"*Raising Adventurous Eaters* provides clinically proven solutions coupled with real-world pragmaticism for parents feeling rudderless in a sea of blue-box macaroni. Lara Dato's wealth of experience in her private practice working with children and families struggling with feeding challenges is carefully composed as a go-to resource for a broad range of picky eating challenges. Mealtime harmony can now be within your family's reach."

> —**Allison Rinehart**, culinary instructor, and
> founder of Lil' Pinkies Up

"Thank you to Lara Dato for finally bringing us a book that dives deep into the relationship between sensory processing and eating with easy-to-understand terminology and practical examples. This book is a wonderful resource for parents, caregivers, feeding therapists, and other health care professionals looking for insight on how to help children with sensory processing challenges learn to eat and explore new foods."

> —**Samantha Goldman, PP-OTD**, CEO of
> Samantha N. Goldman, P.A.; and founder of the
> Food Explorers Membership for parents of children
> with feeding difficulties

"Empowering adventurous eaters through practical, put-in-use-today strategies for families throughout the eight senses. Lara Dato breaks down each sense and offers easy-to-emulate activities and worksheets throughout mealtimes. Her extensive knowledge and experience shine through. A creative and practical guide that will be in my clinic referral resources."

> —**Melissa Longhurst, MS, CCC-SLP**, own
> Advanced Therapy Solutions

"*Raising Adventurous Eaters* takes parents and caretakers on a tour of the senses, explaining how each sense informs eating, how sensory sensitivities may interfere with eating, and how to help kids overcome picky eating so they grow to love all foods. A fresh approach and must-have guide for parents with fussy eaters!"

—**Jill Castle**, pediatric dietitian, founder of
The Nourished Child, author of *Try New Food*
and *Size Wise*, and coauthor of *Fearless Feeding*

"A wonderful and practical resource for families and clinicians. Lara is an expert in her field, with years of experience in treating pediatric feeding. In this book, she provides creative strategies for introducing new foods, managing sensory input, and setting up successful mealtimes. This book is a must for anyone dealing with picky eaters!"

—**Jayme Beal, MS, CCC-SLP**, owner of Rescue My
Speech Pediatric Therapies in Henderson, NV

"Lara Dato's experience and expertise—working with the average picky eater to medically complex children—shine in this thoughtful and novel approach to feeding. It is well organized, easy to read, and contains lots of practical examples. I would highly recommend this book for all parents, no matter the age or stage your child is at!"

—**Kelly Klaczkiewicz, RD, CSP**, pediatric dietitian

RAISING ADVENTUROUS EATERS

Practical Ways to Overcome Picky Eating & Food Sensory Sensitivities

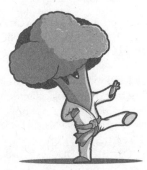

LARA DATO, MS, OTR/L

New Harbinger Publications, Inc.

NEW HARBINGER PUBLICATIONS is a registered trademark of New Harbinger Publications, Inc.

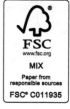

New Harbinger Publications is an employee-owned company.

Copyright © 2022 by Lara Dato
New Harbinger Publications, Inc.
5674 Shattuck Avenue
Oakland, CA 94609
www.newharbinger.com

Cover design by Sara Christian

Acquired by Elizabeth Hollis Hansen

Edited by Joyce Wu

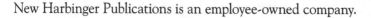

Library of Congress Cataloging-in-Publication Data

Names: Dato, Lara, author.
Title: Raising adventurous eaters : practical ways to overcome picky eating and food sensory sensitivities / by Lara Dato MS OTR/L, SC-FES.
Description: Oakland, CA : New Harbinger Publications, Inc., [2022] | Includes bibliographical references.
Identifiers: LCCN 2022028021 | ISBN 9781684039524 (trade paperback)
Subjects: LCSH: Children--Nutrition--Psychological aspects. | Food preferences in children. | Child psychology. | Child rearing. | BISAC: FAMILY & RELATIONSHIPS / Children with Special Needs | PSYCHOLOGY / Psychopathology / Eating Disorders
Classification: LCC HQ784.E3 D37 2022 | DDC 649/.3--dc23/eng/20220802
LC record available at https://lccn.loc.gov/2022028021

Printed in the United States of America

24   23   22

10   9   8   7   6   5   4   3   2   1   First Printing

Contents

Part Ten: Maintaining Sensory Regulation

Foreword

Picky eating has been around since the dawn of time and has been a frustrating aspect of child-rearing for millions of parents worldwide. The antiquated guidance for parents was typically to force children to eat any and all food that was served to them. Children were told to stay at the table until they ate everything on their plate, sometimes lasting well into the evening. Unfortunately, this harsh approach only made mealtime a battleground, creating long-term damage to family relationships and the relationship between the child and food. Additionally, this approach did not increase a child's willingness or ability to eat a wider variety of foods. Quite the opposite—it created a stressful, if not traumatic, memory around eating in general or eating certain foods.

Parents have longed for some real help, and Lara Dato has delivered. In *Raising Adventurous Eaters*, Dato has created a useful, informational, and easy-to-follow book that provides real-world guidance as to how to help children who are picky eaters, have limited palates, have trouble eating, or don't get proper nutrition from their food intake. Fortunately for the parents, families, and professionals who work with these children, *Raising Adventurous Eaters* is now here.

As two mental health professionals who have written several books about sensory processing issues and how they affect behavior, emotions, and overall health, we have been eager to see more good resources for parents and families who are challenged with these issues. Dato presents the biology of sensory processing in an understandable and normalized way, making the information presented in this book easy to digest and relevant to a wide array of parents, in a supportive and nonjudgmental tone. Picky eating can disrupt the family system. These disruptions can create a tense battleground during mealtimes, affect relationships, and result in hurt and angry feelings. This book is an excellent resource that will change how parents of picky eaters approach meals with their child.

Raising Adventurous Eaters provides tangible ideas to help struggling families approach mealtime differently, which hopefully, when presented at an early age, will prevent these struggles altogether. This book is a guide to healthy eating and peaceful mealtimes for almost any sensory-oriented child. Dato provides an understandable overview of the nervous system and how children with sensory regulation problems may respond to foods that are hard for their nervous systems to manage. She outlines not only the five near senses (smell, touch, sight, taste, and sound), but also the three far senses (interoceptive, proprioceptive, and vestibular) as they relate to food, eating, and mealtime behavior. In addition, Dato then gives specific instructions to parents about how to change mealtime environments to make the introduction of food more palatable to children who have very particular sensory sensitivities.

Sensory processing and how it can impact children, childhood behavior, and childhood emotional functioning has long been underrepresented and underappreciated in literature. We're so excited to see this book, with such a wealth of information, concrete ideas, and emotional support, become available to parents in need. We wish we had read this book when our children were young!

Raising a child with sensory processing issues can be challenging, but this book is a life-saver for parents struggling to successfully feed their child. This book will be widely recommended by both of us to our clients struggling in this arena. Hats off to Lara Dato for providing so many ideas and suggestions to parents about how to help persnickety eaters. By having insight about what might trigger these negative responses to food, parents and caretakers are able to provide interesting and appealing solutions, creating a healthy, happy mealtime environment for the entire family.

—Suzanne Mouton-Odum, PhD, and
Ruth Goldfinger Golomb, LCPC

Clinicians and Coauthors of *Helping Your Child with Sensory Regulation*

Introduction

If you know and love a young picky eater, you're not alone! Recent studies show that 25–45 percent of typically developing children have trouble with eating, and that number shoots up to 80 percent for children with any other health condition (Bryant-Waugh et al. 2010). Having trouble with eating is incredibly common, but that doesn't mean you have to live with it.

As a feeding therapist and lover of many picky eaters myself, I've seen firsthand how picky eating can affect your entire family. Food and mealtimes are huge parts of bonding with family and friends, of participating in and learning about culture, and of exploring the world around us. Eating is something we do three to six times a day, which means that when it's going poorly, there's going to be a lot of extra stress in your day.

Positive mealtime experiences are essential: they set both you and your child up for a successful day. Getting the right nutrients readies your child to learn and participate in all the other areas of development that they want to focus on, like running, reading, playing with friends, and more. When picky eating prevents your child from getting all of the foods that they need, you spend more time stressing and less time doing the things that you and your child love to do! The sooner you address your concerns around your child's eating, the sooner you can get on to enjoyable and stress-free mealtimes for the whole family.

As you embark on the journey of encouraging adventurous eating, know that although eating seems simple, it's actually one of the most complex things we do as humans. Eating requires using all our body systems, all our senses, and dozens of muscles. To eat, children need to:

- Move their cheek muscles, lips, and tongue to chew and move food in their mouth.

- Coordinate their breathing with their chewing and swallowing.

- Do all this while processing and learning about new sensory experiences with the tastes and smells of new foods.

That's a lot to tie together! There's a big misconception that children are born knowing how to eat. This is somewhat true up until six months old. Children are born with reflexes that help them drink breastmilk or formula. These reflexes disappear by the time they're six months old though, just in time to start eating solid foods. After this, every eating skill needs to be learned, and none of them come naturally.

As a parent, you have a vital role in the acquisition of these skills. When left to their own devices, picky eaters often fall further into their restrictive habits. Children that feel uncertain about trying new foods typically avoid new foods altogether, causing a downward spiral into even pickier eating habits. As a parent, you can act as a tour guide in their journey toward adventurous eating. You can prepare them with the techniques and confidence that they'll need for a lifetime of positive eating habits. No matter when you take the first steps on this journey, it's never too late to get started.

If the picky-eating woes have you feeling down right now, don't give up hope. There's much you can do to support your child in growing into an adventurous eater. Backed by science and a long history of helping families just like yours, this book will guide you through the what, how, and why of making changes to help your picky eater grow and develop.

What Is Sensory Processing?

Sensory processing is how the body organizes sensation from one's own body and the environment, making it possible to use the body effectively within the environment. Our bodies use our sensory systems to interpret the world around us and help us make sense of it. When we think of our sensory systems, we typically think of the five most talked about systems: our sight, smell, touch, taste, and hearing. In actuality, there are three more senses: Our *proprioceptive sense* helps us figure out where our body is in space and plan our movements, while our *vestibular sense* is our sense of balance. Last, our *interoceptive sense* gives us information about what's going on inside our bodies. It tells us when we're hungry, when we're full, when we're thirsty, when we need to go to the bathroom, and so much more.

All of these senses work together to help our bodies understand our world (and our food!). For each one, we get input from our environment every second of every day. We hear and see things around us, feel everything we touch, smell our environment, taste everything that goes in our mouths, hear people talking to us, feel our bodies moving, sense how we're balanced, and feel what's going on inside our bodies. All of our sensory systems work together constantly to help us function throughout our day, and we use every single one of these senses while eating.

You can think of our sensory preferences as a sliding scale from zero to one hundred, with each person occupying a particular position on the scale, reflecting their unique preferences on the amount of input that their body gets. For the purposes of this metaphor, you could say that the average person has a preference of somewhere between forty to sixty, but everybody is different. Some people prefer lots of input (between eighty and one hundred), and some people prefer less input (between zero and twenty). I like to think of the ideal zone each of us has as our "sweet spot." When our levels of input match our body's preferences—when they're in our sweet spot—we do our best learning and engaging.

A good example of this is how listening to music—using our auditory sense—helps or distracts from learning. Some people need a quiet library to study efficiently, while others put headphones on and need music to stay focused. The people who prefer no background noise might prefer lower amounts of input, while people who prefer loud music have a higher input-zone preference. Neither way of processing auditory input is better or worse, but they change the way that we explore our world. Each of our senses has similar differences.

In addition to having unique preferences within one sense, we all have different preferences for each one of our senses. One person may enjoy high amounts of auditory input, but prefer lower amounts of visual input.

Because each sense preference is different, you need to look at each sense independently to know how your child functions best.

How a Sensory Processing Approach Can Help

Eating (and learning to love new foods) can be difficult because it challenges every one of our senses. Biting into a new food bombards our senses with information. Our bodies simultaneously smell, taste, feel, and see our food while hearing our bites crunching. They also need to coordinate all the movements for sitting and chewing. That's a lot of information to receive and organize all at once! Using a sensory-based approach to exploring food helps your child's body process all that sensory information in the most productive way possible.

Using this approach, you'll learn more about how your child's body uniquely processes the world around it, and you'll be able to individualize strategies to set them up for success. Because everyone's bodies experience the world a little differently, strategies for learning how to eat are not a one-size-fits-all method. This book's approach takes these individualities into account and provides personalized techniques to best support your learning eater as they experience the world of food.

Because they're still learning about their bodies, your child likely won't be able to articulate their own sensory preferences. Parents need to be detectives in figuring out their child's sensory needs and preferences. To start making sense of the way that your child's body processes food, let's begin by finding any patterns that might exist in their preferences. Doing this will allow you to start to see where their sensory systems may be more comfortable, and in which ways you can support them with more challenging foods. The following activity will help you generate information to be used later on in the book. You can either visit http://www.newharbinger .com/49524 to download the worksheet (and other free tools) or use a piece of paper to consider the following questions:

- What are your child's top ten favorite foods?

- What do those foods look like? What colors are they? How big are the typical serving sizes?

- What are the textures of those foods? Do those textures change as you chew them? For example, a grape may feel dry and firm to the touch, but the texture may be wet and juicy as you chew it.

- What do those foods smell like?

- What do those foods taste like?

- What do those foods sound like when you chew them? Are they crunchy or chewy?

- Does your child have a favorite place to eat? Will they only eat if walking or wiggling around, or do they sit still at the table?

As you fill out these questions, do you notice any patterns starting to emerge? For example, maybe your child only likes crunchy foods, or maybe they prefer foods that are bland in color. Keep these patterns and preferences in mind as you read the rest of this book. The later chapters will help you make sense of these patterns and help you use them to guide your child's eating journey. You can use these patterns and preferences to link their current favorite foods with foods that they haven't yet learned to like.

While everyone is born with sensory preferences, a lot can influence those preferences. On a day-to-day basis, our preferences can change based on our sleep, nutrition, pain, and overall health. To go back to our example of music, someone that loves loud music on an average day may become frustrated by music played too loudly on a day when they're exhausted, hungry, or in pain.

The ways our bodies function outside of our sensory preference zones can also change over time, as can our sensory preference zones themselves, with intentional practice and positive experiences. With the tools and practices I'll share in this book, you can help set your child up for success by individualizing their learning experiences with food. You'll explore how their body and sensory systems learn best, and discover ways to incorporate these into their mealtime routines. These strategies will help limit your child's tantrums, irritability, and anxiety around trying new foods. You can support your child in creating positive associations with experiences slightly outside their ideal sensory zones. This can help your child learn to tolerate, and feel comfortable and confident with, different sensory experiences. And soon, you'll have an enthusiastic eater that's eager to come to the table.

How Sensory Processing Affects Eating

Eating new foods can be a huge challenge for each of our senses. Children use their senses to understand and make sense of a new food long before it ever reaches their mouth. Children often use all their senses to learn about a food before eating it:

- When it's first presented to them, they'll look at it and smell it.

- They'll touch it with a utensil or their fingers.

- They'll bring it up to their face, where they can better smell it or touch it to their lips or tongue.

- They may watch other people eat it and listen to how chewing it sounds.

- After building up confidence with all these steps, they may feel more ready to take their first bite.

As you may be all too aware, if anything stirs discomfort along the way, children may refuse a new food entirely. Children use these sensory explorations to prepare for taking a bite. As they're looking at, smelling, and touching food, they're making preliminary guesses about what the experience of eating it may be like. If they're uncomfortable with what the food looked like, or how it felt on their fingers, they're highly unlikely to feel confident about exploring the food further. This can feel frustrating and daunting to parent and child alike. As an adult, watching a child refuse a food can look like a split-second refusal, without any consideration for the food itself. After all, you've likely spent time buying ingredients for, preparing, and serving this food to your child, all to have them immediately refuse it. From the child's perspective though, their senses *have* given them information—and they're likely experiencing a sense of deep uncertainty and worry about what they're being asked to eat. They're also noticing that they're under pressure to eat something that their instincts are telling them to avoid. The key is to empower them with the knowledge and strategies that they need to feel comfortable with a new food, and to help them develop the new preferences that you're hoping they'll adopt.

Children use all their senses to explore food, so to introduce new foods, we need to understand how each sense affects their learning and exploration. To understand how these senses work together, let's first look at each sense alone and how it affects mealtime routines. After you read about each sense, pause to consider the information that you gathered through the questionnaire you filled out earlier. As you read, you'll learn more about your child's own ideal preference zone for each sense.

Sight. For many children, this is the first sense that they use to examine a new food. What does the food look like? What color is it? What size is it? Does it look wet or dry? There are so many things they can tell just by looking at a food. Many children decide that a food looks "safe" or "unsafe" just by its visual appearance.

Children who prefer *higher levels of visual input* tend to prefer bright colors and busy backgrounds. They tend to do better with having brightly colored foods or having several foods on their plates together. Children who prefer *lower levels of visual input* tend to prefer blander colors and fewer visual distractions. These children may gravitate toward foods that are white or tan in color, or may be very specific about having minimal amounts and volumes of foods on their plates.

Touch. Next, your child may be willing to touch a new food. What does the food feel like? Is it wet or dry? Rough or smooth? Does it leave any residue on their fingers? Children explore foods with their fingers to understand what the texture is like before they're ready to see what it will feel like in their mouths. This is why toddlers tend to be such messy eaters. When they bang a carrot against their high chair, they're learning that the carrot is hard and they'll have to bite down hard. When they run purees through their hair, they're feeling if there are any chunks that they may have to munch on before swallowing. The feeling of food in their hands indicates what that food will feel like in their mouth, and touching food is their way of learning about the texture.

A child who prefers *high amounts of tactile input* is likely a messy eater. They'll like eating with their fingers and won't mind or notice the food on their skin. You may have to remind them to use a napkin or clean off their mouth after eating, because their body may not notice that it's messy. A child who prefers *low amounts of tactile input* will be hypervigilant about keeping themselves clean. They may be reluctant to pick up their food or may cry if their hands get messy. Take a moment to consider your child's tactile sensory preferences and review what you filled out on the "Touch" section of the online worksheet or your piece of paper.

Smell. After touching a food, we next use our sense of smell to determine more about it. Our sense of smell correlates with some of our strongest memories. Many of us remember walking into a family member's house and smelling a favorite family recipe in the kitchen. Our children associate smells with food experiences as well. Does it smell sweet or savory? Does it smell similar to a food they've had before, or is it a whole new smell? Smelling a food can be a wonderful way to explore it before actually tasting it.

A child who prefers *low amounts of input to their smell sense* may prefer foods without much odor, while children that prefer *high input* may lean toward spicier or "smellier" foods. Take a moment to consider your child's ideal smell sensory preferences and review what you filled out on the "Smell" section of the online worksheet or your piece of paper.

Taste. Most adults associate food with taste, but it's typically one of the last senses that children use to explore their food. Children will likely look at, smell, and touch a food before even giving it a taste. Children have preferences for taste just like adults do. They may prefer bland or spicy, sweet or savory, fruity or grainy.

Children who prefer *low amounts of taste input* will gravitate toward blander foods, like crackers, breads, and chicken nuggets. They may become upset if you put sauce or seasoning on their food. Children who like *higher amounts of input* prefer more flavorful or spicy foods. These children may enjoy putting spices or sauces on their food. They may like using dips to make their foods more flavorful. If they feel like their food isn't flavorful enough, they might put more food in their mouth so that they can have a stronger taste. Take a moment to consider your child's ideal taste sensory preferences and review what you filled out on the "Taste" section of the online worksheet or your piece of paper.

Hearing. It may seem odd that our auditory sense would have anything to do with food, but for children, it can be a great learning and exploration tool. When they put a food in their mouth, what does it sound like—a slurp or a crunch?

Children who prefer *low amounts of auditory input* may become frustrated by the sound of people chewing or talking at the dinner table. They may become overwhelmed by sound, and this could show through reluctance to sit at the table, frequent tantrums, or refusal to eat around other people. Children who prefer *higher amounts of auditory input* may like crunchy foods and loud noises, and may talk loudly at the dining table. Take a moment to consider your child's auditory sensory preferences and review what you filled out on the "Hearing" section of the online worksheet or your piece of paper.

Proprioception. Our proprioceptive sense is our sense of body awareness. It helps us know where our body is in space and helps us plan motor movements. It helps us know where food is in our mouth and tells us how to string together the movements of putting a food in our mouth, chewing, and swallowing. It also tells us how hard we need to chew to be able to break a food down into a texture that we can swallow.

We get the information for our proprioceptive system from our muscles, joints, and skin. Foods that are harder in texture, or require more pressure to chew, give us more proprioceptive input. This means that it's easier to tell where a hard food is in our mouth than it is a soft food.

Sometimes when children have lower levels of body awareness, they may shove more food in their mouth or leave food in their mouth rather than immediately swallow it. The more food there is in our mouth, the more pressure it puts on our mouth, and the more proprioceptive input we receive. Children who prefer *higher amounts of proprioceptive input* tend to prefer harder or crunchier foods, and children who prefer *lower amounts of proprioceptive input* may prefer softer foods, even if they're physically capable of eating harder foods. Children who prefer higher amounts of proprioceptive input are often described as "on-the-go," or they may enjoy active, rough play. Children who prefer lower amounts of proprioceptive input may prefer more sedentary play. Take a moment to consider your child's proprioceptive preferences, given what you know about their preferred play styles and preferred foods and bite size.

Vestibular. Our vestibular system is our balance system. It tells us how our head is attached to our body: Are we leaning forward? To the side? Backward? This is very important for the positioning of children while they eat. The safest eating position for a child is one where they're sitting upright, with their hips, knees, and ankles at a ninety-degree angle. We want their backs and feet to be supported. With a well-balanced and well-supported position, our children are at less risk to choke. They're also more likely to remain focused at the table. They're more engaged with their food and learning about food, and this sets them up for success in trying new foods. Take a moment to consider the position of your child while they're seated at the table.

Interoception. Our interoception helps us know and understand what's going on inside our body. It's actually one of the most important sensory systems that we have! It tells us when we're hungry and when we're full. It tells us when we're thirsty, when we're in pain, when we're hot, and when we're cold. Children are still learning about their bodies, and can sometimes misinterpret the signals that their interoceptive sense is giving them. For example, they may not yet understand the difference between a belly ache, hunger pangs, pressure from a full stomach, and the sensation of butterflies in their stomach from anxiety. Many children confuse or misascribe different types of abdominal discomfort, which could cause them to misunderstand stomach fullness for a belly ache caused by sickness. If this happens, they may worry that they're making themselves sick every time they eat a large meal.

Other forces, like constipation and reflux, can scramble those signals. When children are constipated, they tend to eat less. There's simply less room in their digestive system, as it's blocked by an unpassed bowel movement, which their body processes as, "I'm not hungry yet," even if it's their scheduled meal time. Reflux can also impact appetite. If eating typically results in discomfort associated with reflux, their body may learn to pair eating with discomfort, decreasing their desire to eat.

Although all our sensory systems work together, everyone has different preferences for each one of our systems, and this can affect our food preferences. No two people have exactly the same sensory preferences.

As adults, we understand our preferences and modify our behavior so that we can complete our daily tasks efficiently. If a food is too spicy, we may take a drink between bites, or we may take smaller bites. If a food is too bland, we may mix it with other foods that are already on our plate, or add a sauce. We may even do this subconsciously. Adapting their behavior can be much harder for children, as they're still learning about their bodies.

Exploring new foods is much like adventuring through anything new: sometimes it can be scary, but we can succeed with confidence. Understanding their sensory preferences will help your child feel more comfortable with new sensory food experiences, which will in turn help you create positive experiences that empower your children and let them know they can take on anything, inside the dining room and out.

To take the stress off both you and your child, make sure not to call them a picky eater. If you label your child as a picky eater, they may internalize that. Instead, we want to empower them to feel like strong and brave eaters. Support your child and be excited with them when they try a new food. Sometimes the steps to becoming an adventurous eater can feel small, but lots of small steps together make for big leaps. If you support their little victories and validate them when they take positive steps, your child will soon see themselves as an adventurous eater.

How to Use This Book

Now that you have a better sense of your child's preferred levels of **sensory input**—the stimulation of their senses—let's talk about how this book can help you support your child's sensory systems for successful eating.

Of course, for a complete experience, you can read this book from cover to cover. This book is organized by sense, with strategies for each sensory experience that your child will have when trying a new food. The order of chapters models the natural sensory exploration process that your child may go through, starting with looking at the food for the first time and progressing through touching it, smelling it, tasting it, and hearing their first bites. Then the book will provide you with strategies for improving your child's body awareness and positioning around eating. Finally, it wraps up with strategies for supporting your child's mental health, body image, and overall regulation and well-being around food.

If, while filling out your child's sensory questionnaire, you noticed any particular patterns, you may want to target your reading to the sections related to the senses that your child is having difficulty with. For example, if your child only eats foods that are tan or white, you may have identified that their visual system is a sensory system that's limiting their food preferences. In that case, you may want to jump immediately to the chapters on vision for on-the-spot help, later circling back to the other senses to see how it all ties together.

To support you on your adventurous eating journey, I've developed a series of worksheets and activities that you can find on New Harbinger's website for this book: http://www.newharbinger.com/49524 These pages will be referenced throughout the book, with prompts and suggested activities. Feel free to look them up as you go along or print them all out as you start the book so that you have them ready to complete.

Ultimately, I've found the sensory-based approach this book elaborates on to be highly effective in my clinical practice for children of all ages. With this approach, I've helped countless children and their families transition from stressful mealtimes and picky eating to relaxed meals, full of connection, love, and of course, adventurous eating! As you read, it's likely various principles—those crucial to ending mealtime battles for control and to raising an adventurous eater who's curious about and confident with food—will become clear. And these principles will become even easier to experience and master as you begin experimenting with the strategies that seem most helpful for you and your child. In case you come across a term that seems unfamiliar, I've included a glossary at the end of the book.

Regardless of how you choose to experience this book, the strategies in here will set you and your child up for a lifetime of success in the dining room!

Part One

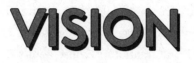

VISION

Have you ever heard the phrase "You eat with your eyes first"? We gain so much information based on the appearance of food before we ever bring it to our mouths. As adults, we can look at a food and know so much about it. We can look at it and decide what it'll feel like in our mouths. We can know if it'll be chewy, crunchy, or soft. Its appearance can tell us if and how we'll have to chew it before swallowing it. That's a ton of information!

Now consider it from your child's perspective. Their first experience with a new food is also looking at it. But looking at a food doesn't give them nearly so much information. Because adults have had many, many more years of experience and time to learn, children simply don't have the same repertoire.

These limitations can be even more extreme for picky eaters, some of whom avoid even looking at new foods because it makes them anxious. That's why one of the first steps toward learning to love a new food is becoming comfortable looking at it!

Some learning eaters form incorrect assumptions about the appearance of food and how it correlates with taste. For example, consider a child who has eaten a very limited number of red foods. Let's say they've eaten strawberries, raspberries, and red grapes. They may assume that all red foods are juicy and sweet, because in their experience, that's true. Now this child goes to eat another red food, like a red pepper, but it's spicy and not sweet! This is completely unexpected, and now they're feeling very unsure. Feelings of anxiety and confusion are counterproductive to eating and trying new foods.

To learn more about your child's visual preferences in relation to foods, look at your log of all the foods that they're willing to eat. Are there any trends in food appearance? For example, some children only eat white or tan foods, like chicken nuggets, breads, and pastas. Some children are picky about their foods touching, and want them all separate on the plate. Some picky eaters can be easily overwhelmed by the visual appearance of new foods and try to avoid looking at new or non-preferred foods when possible. Knowing about your child's visual preferences can help you to set their meals up for success.

The good news about our visual sense is that we can modify how a food looks to make it feel "safer." As you read through this section, you'll gain tips for how to do this, such as cutting foods up into small bites, putting less of it on a plate, or even covering it in sauce to change its color. Smaller serving sizes and bite sizes can make a food look less visually overwhelming, and colors can inspire your child to try it before rejecting it.

Supporting your child's visual sense allows them to feel confident and secure during mealtimes. From the way you present and plate food, to how you introduce it, there are many ways to set adventurous eating up for success. In this chapter, we'll cover ways to:

- Introduce new foods by appealing to your child's visual sense.

- Adjust the way you plate and serve dinner, so your child can participate in food preparation and get more used to food.

- Help your child diversify the brands of food they're willing to try—especially if they've latched on to one brand they like.

- Help your child stay focused on the mealtime and learning about new foods, without being distracted by what's going on around the house.

- Make mealtimes fun and visually appealing!

1   Introducing New Foods

Introducing your child to new foods can be one of the most fun parts of raising an adventurous eater, but it can be frustrating to meet with resistance. We all look forward to sharing our favorite foods and building those memories of cooking and tasting, and there are lots of strategies that you can use to make sure your child has successful experiences with new foods.

When you're offering new foods, it's typically best to offer only one new food at a time, ideally served with something that you know your child likes. If you offer too many new foods at once, your child may feel overwhelmed and therefore shut down. We want our children to feel confident and adventurous, and offering just one new food at a time can help them feel this way.

To support your child in using their visual sense to explore their food, make sure you're exposing them to foods that are all the colors of the rainbow. This can start as soon as you introduce them to their very first foods as a baby. Offer them a very small amount (pea-sized). They can always ask for more. Offering less of a new food will make it appear easier to manage from a visual standpoint and will increase the odds of their being willing to try it.

Another thing to keep in mind before starting to introduce a new food is that it can take a child up to twenty exposures to a new food before they can make an accurate decision about whether or not they like that food (Carruth and Skinner 2000). This means that you may need to offer your child the same food twenty times before they're willing to eat it. I know that twenty exposures sounds like a *ton*, and that can feel daunting. Many parents expect their child to taste (and ideally, enjoy) a food the first time they're offered it, but in reality, very few children will do this. They need repeated opportunities to interact with the food so they can learn about it. A large part of their learning process is becoming comfortable with the food with their visual system, and then tying that to their other sensory systems. They need to learn about what it looks like, smells like, and feels like on their hands and lips before they're going to be willing to try tasting it. From an evolutionary perspective, spending so much time learning about your food before eating it is a safe choice. While it can feel like a lot of work to offer your child so many learning opportunities, remember that each time you offer your child a food, you are helping them move one step closer to adding that food to their normal *food repertoire*, or the list of foods that your child is willing to eat.

To create opportunities for exposures to new foods, you want to create an environment where your child can interact with the food. There are tons of ways to do this before you even make it to the kitchen. Have your child help at the grocery store, farmer's market, or in the garden. There, they can learn about all sorts of foods and start to prepare for what they might taste like. Produce can be especially anxiety inducing for picky eaters, as fruits and vegetables vary so much in appearance. Use the grocery store as a place to empower your child with knowledge about these foods. Teach them how to tell when a food is ripe versus unripe and how it tastes different over time. This will help them learn to identify what new foods will taste like based on their visual appearance.

You can also have them help in the kitchen with cooking and baking. Children make great sous chefs, so have them help with the mixing, pouring, and sorting. They'll get a chance to start building up exposures and experiences with food before mealtime. What's more, many foods change appearances while cooking—for example, spinach can be bright green and leafy before cooking, and dark green and wilted after cooking— and without experience, you may not even know that these are the same food! Having your child help in the kitchen can strengthen their knowledge of food appearances so they feel more comfortable tasting it.

You can continue to support their exploration at the dining table too. When exposed to new food, children can hesitate. Some children may try to limit themselves to just looking at the food, but as a parent, you can help your child become more comfortable with the food by encouraging them to play with or otherwise interact with it. As a family, you can talk about what it looks or smells like. You could have your child help stir the food using a utensil, or they could practice poking the food with a toothpick or fork. Your child can help serve their siblings and can help clean up their plate. All of these experiences allow your child to learn about the food with their eyes. As children become more comfortable with unfamiliar or non-preferred foods, they become more likely to try and take a bite.

Children learn best from the people they love the most—their parents! If your child sees you eating and participating in mealtime routines, they're likely to want to copy you. You can set a good example for your child by being a good role model. Try all the foods that you want your child to try. If you don't eat a food, your child won't either. It can help to talk about and really sell the food. Children are significantly more likely to eat a food if they watch you eat it with a positive expression on your face (Edwards et al. 2022). If you look like you're having fun and enjoying it, your child may wonder what they're missing out on and want to try too. Parents that are picky eaters teach their children to be picky eaters by example, and parents that are adventurous eaters inspire their children to be adventurous as well.

To create a family routine that supports adventurous eaters, serve your meals family style, with all the foods set out in the center of the table for people to serve themselves from. With the foods all already on the table, your child will have more of an opportunity to interact with those foods, even if they aren't ready to eat them just yet. Depending on their age, your child can be responsible for helping serve everyone at the table. By spooning the food onto everyone's plates (or even just their own), they'll have an opportunity to interact more mindfully with the food and to consider the appearance, texture, and smell before it even reaches their plate.

Also set the expectation that everyone put at least one spoonful of each food on their plate. If your child is unsure, just remind them, "In our family, we take a little bit of every food." I say "a little bit" rather than "a bite" of every food, because the expectation is not necessarily that your child has to eat every food every time it's on their plate. Rather, we want to give them the experience interacting with the food so that they feel comfortable trying it on their own. Forcing children to eat can create anxiety and make them feel opposed to trying a new food. With ample opportunities to interact with the food, they'll feel empowered to try it on their own, without pressure.

To this end, I recommend having a larger serving spoon and a small tasting spoon that is around the size of a half-teaspoon or smaller. When it comes to each food, ask your child if they would like a big spoonful or a little spoonful. With preferred foods, they may choose a big spoonful, and with new foods, a little spoonful. The serving size of the little spoonful should be around the size of a pea. Smaller serving sizes will make your child more likely to try a new food because they'll feel less pressure and anxiety around it. When we offer a child a large amount of food, it comes with an implicit pressure (whether we voice this or not) for them to eat the entire amount. That can feel too scary, so rather than try a little bit of it and feel pressured to eat the whole thing, they'll avoid the food altogether. When we offer a very small, pea-sized amount, the child will be much more willing to try tasting it. They may like it and ask for more!

It's good to remember to keep serving sizes of their favorite foods to a small or moderate size. If we fill up their plate with their favorite food, they're likely to eat and fill up on that, leaving no room for the new food. Of course, your child can always ask for seconds or thirds of their favorite food, but serving a smaller initial portion can motivate them to try the new food too. Children are much more likely to try a new food if they aren't already filled up with their favorite food.

Your child is most likely to try a new food when they're a little bit hungry. Of course, we never want to starve our children, but children who have totally full stomachs aren't very likely to feel motivated to try a new food. If your child is starving, they may just want familiar foods, but if they're just a little hungry, they may be ready to try new things. It takes about two hours for food to clear from a child's stomach, so it can be helpful to limit their food intake for about two hours prior to feeding them a meal that contains a new food. Picking mealtimes when your child is ready to eat will help encourage them to sample all the foods on their plate, including unfamiliar ones.

Many of us adults were raised with a "You have to eat everything on your plate" policy, and it can feel tempting to apply the same policy in our children's lives. For many picky children though, this can backfire instead. For starters, such a policy teaches our children to judge their fullness based on what's left on their plate rather than how their body feels. It can lead to their having less understanding of their body cues as they get older, and can lead to an unhealthy relationship with food. Studies show that children who are forced to eat everything on their plates are more likely to use food as a coping strategy as they get older and are more likely to be overweight (Pfeffer 2009; Robinson and Hardman 2016). Forcing your child to eat everything on their plate also sets up a battle that you aren't likely to win. Trying to force your child to eat something can turn it into a bigger fight than it needs to be, and can turn them off of that food. Your child is more likely to develop mindfulness and confidence around food if they can listen to their body cues to decide when they're done eating.

There are lots of strategies to introduce your child to new foods, but it's okay if it takes time. Don't take your child's refusal personally. It's 100 percent normal to be wary of trying new foods. By using the strategies outlined in this chapter, you can set up your child up for success when introducing them to new foods. Trying new foods will soon be something fun to look forward to rather than a stressor or something to be nervous about.

2 Plates and Plating

Choosing the right plate and arranging the food on it in a way that sets your child up for success can be key for supporting your child's visual system. There are several different types of plates that you can consider for your child.

Some children with preferences for higher visual input are very motivated by plates with decorations or pictures on them. It can be especially exciting for children if they have an opportunity to pick out their own "fun plate." Choosing their own special plate can increase their feelings of investment toward their meals. If your child uses a plate with a favorite character or animal on it, they may be motivated to look at their food or clear their plate. They learn that, by eating their food, they can reveal a picture or image that they're excited about.

For children who are fussy if their foods touch, you can buy plates that have divided sections.

If your child likes trying to throw their plate, they may benefit from a plate with suction on the bottom. Suction plates and bowls come in a variety of shapes and colors, and can really cut down on potential throwing and mess.

If your child is young enough to be in a high chair, they may not need a plate at all. Putting food directly on their tray allows you to spread the food out further, which may help pace them and keep them more mindful of their food. Doing this also eliminates any distraction that may be caused by a plate.

Regardless of which type of plate you choose for your child, it can help to have a couple different options and to let your child choose which plate they want to use at each meal. Having control is so important to increasing their investment in the meal, and allowing them to pick out their plate will increase their willingness to adventure with new food.

Once you have the right plate for your child, you can start to think about how you want to present their food.

We live in the age of the internet and social media, and who hasn't seen parents share pictures of the artfully plated meal they've created for their child? There are parents creating entire scenes made out of just food to get their child to eat, and to present a certain image to the world. Does that really make a difference in children's food intake? While it can be fun and novel for a short while, in the long term, it's likely that the answer is no. And beyond that, who has time to create a masterpiece several times a day? Certainly not me!

Research actually shows that children through preteen years prefer deconstructed meals, or meals where each ingredient is separate from the others (Zampollo et al. 2012). For example, on taco night, you would serve the ingredients—tortilla, meat, other toppings—in separate piles on the plate rather than all together. This preference for deconstructed meals makes complete sense! Children are still learning about new foods, and having each food separate allows them to learn about each food individually, rather than feel overwhelmed by too many flavor combinations at once. It also makes it easy for children to see which foods they're going to be putting in their mouth with each bite, as opposed to a mixed food, like a taco, where one bite may have a lot of one particular topping that isn't easily discernable by taste alone.

In addition to the way to plate children's foods, families often feel a lot of pressure to preload their children's plates with food. Children actually do better and eat more if they're allowed to serve themselves though. Family-style meals, where family members take turns serving themselves, allow your child to take more control over and responsibility for their food intake. As I described in the last chapter, I typically recommend having a small spoon and a large spoon in each food, which allows your child to choose if they'd like a small spoonful or a large spoonful of each type of food. Using two spoons ensures that they get at least a little bit of everything on their plate while empowering them to actively participate in their food choices. It also makes sure that they don't get an overwhelming amount of a non-preferred food on their plate.

Children, especially those who prefer less visual input, can feel overwhelmed by large servings of foods that they're unsure about, and when this happens, they're less likely to try them. They tend to be more likely to try a new food if there's only a small quantity of it on their plate, rather than a large one. A small quantity doesn't overwhelm our visual system in the same way that a large one does.

At first your child might be reluctant to choose which size spoon they want to use for their least favorite foods. You might get some pushback along the lines of, "I don't want to have *any* of that food!" These are times to stick firm to your new family expectation and to make sure that everyone in the family follows the same rules. If your child remains steadfast in their desire not to choose a serving size, you can offer that they make a different choice: would they like to choose their serving spoon size themselves or would they like you to do it? Most times they'll decide to make their own choice. If they continue to refuse to make a choice, or decide that they would like you to choose their serving size, I recommend choosing the small serving spoon size for them. Ultimately, we want to set them up for success and increase their buy-in to mealtimes.

Allowing your child to participate in these food choices teaches them to listen to their appetite and introduces the idea of what constitutes a healthy meal. If you feel creatively driven and want to artistically (or not so artistically) arrange their food, find a way to incorporate your child into that activity. Maybe you can each decorate your own plate, or you can have a plating competition.

I often find that parents' desire to plate their children's food comes down to control. They want to control their child's portion size in an effort to get them to eat more. Remember that control is important to your child too. They'll be more likely to try new foods if they feel like they had a role to play in that, rather than if they feel like it was all your choice. Allowing your child to arrange the food on their plate is an easy way to give them some autonomy, and to empower them to feel more confident in their food choices.

3   Brand Specificity

"I want yogurt! No, not that yogurt, the one with the monkey on it!" Does that sound familiar? It's very common for picky eaters to latch on to one brand or restaurant that they know they like and refuse to accept anything else. Even if it's the exact same food, they've memorized the visual presentation of that packaging, and familiarity creates a feeling of security for them. This is tricky though, because it can really limit the variety that your child is willing to eat. And what happens if the company redesigns their packaging? You're back to square one.

To help prevent children from getting stuck on the visual presentation of specific brands in the first place, try unpackaging foods before serving them. Removing the food from the eye-catching wrapper and placing it on a regular plate or bowl is helpful for a number of purposes. First, it eliminates the concern for brand specificity entirely. It prevents your child from associating a preferred food with a specific brand, so they learn, "I like yogurt" instead of, "I like the yogurt with the monkey on it."

Second, it helps limit the power of these foods. Advertising is meant to be eye catching. After all, advertising is a multibillion-dollar industry specifically designed to sell more product and make more money. These packages are designed to catch your child's interest and make them ask for that food specifically. Serving the food with the packaging draws special attention to that packaging. It makes the child notice that food more than other foods that don't come in fancy packaging, and gives that food more power. When you serve a packaged food alongside other, nonpackaged foods, it makes that food seem more exciting and thrilling, and it's hard for the other foods to keep up!

If your child has already developed some brand-specific preferences, there's still lots to be done to break down that rigidity. For example, say your child *loves* chicken nuggets but will only eat them from one specific fast-food restaurant. You find yourself going there often because you know they're more likely to eat that than what you prepare at home.

Instead of catering to these preferences and presenting the food exactly as they want, make slow changes to the visual presentation of their preferred meal. For instance, instead of serving chicken nuggets in their carton, start by bringing the carton to the table and putting it on a plate. Once they're comfortable with that, try emptying the carton onto the plate in front of your child. Then, eventually, empty it further away, maybe in the kitchen or elsewhere out of sight. Once your child is comfortable with the food being plated without their preferred packaging and away from their line of sight, you can start to introduce the same food but from different brands, or that you have cooked yourself.

By taking little steps to change the visual appearance of your child's food, you can help break them away from the enticing power of advertising and help them find the joy in the taste and exploration of new foods!

4 Minimizing Visual Distractions

During mealtimes you want your child to focus on their food. Staying focused helps them to learn and supports lifelong adventurous eating habits. Having a visual distraction, like a movie or an iPad, can be helpful in the short term in getting children to try new foods. In the long term though, it actually contributes to picky eating.

Think about when you eat popcorn at the movie theater. If you start munching during the trailers, half your popcorn may be gone before the movie even starts. You aren't aware of how much food you've eaten during that time, but rather you've gone on autopilot. And what did you really consciously think about while you were eating? Did you notice the texture or even the taste of the popcorn? Or was it gone before you realized it? All too often, distractions cause us to tune out of food experiences.

Children who become accustomed to having a distraction while trying new foods can come to rely on this. Even if they'll eat a food while they're distracted, they typically won't eat it without the distraction. While they're watching a screen, they aren't looking at their food. They aren't learning about the appearance, texture, or taste. This reinforces picky eating habits and limits children in eating opportunities away from their preferred distraction. In the long term, having a visual distraction ultimately causes more problems than it solves.

It's important to be mindful while you're at the dining table. This means unplugging. Turn off your iPad, your TV, and your phone and focus on the interactions that you can have with family around the table. Mealtimes are about so much more than just food. They're a chance for your child to learn social skills, to learn about their culture, and to learn about family. If you or your child plugs into electronics while eating, you aren't able to get the full mealtime experience. Children that are focused on a screen or toy are thinking about that item rather than their meal.

They aren't focused on interacting with or exploring new foods—they're just focused on their toy.

Ultimately, children are still learning about food and their bodies. They're learning about how to chew food and what it feels like when their bodies are hungry or satisfied. To go back to our movie theater popcorn example, when we're focused on the movie, we aren't thinking about how much food volume we've eaten. As adults, this may not be the healthiest or most mindful way to eat, but it also isn't as harmful as it is for children. When children are focused on a screen or toy or some other visual distraction, they aren't able to learn the vital things they need to learn about eating, not to mention the cultural and social components of mealtime. Make sure both you and your child unplug during mealtimes, and you'll all get more out of the experience.

If your child depends on distraction, there are a couple different approaches to help wean them off of it.

Weaning off a visual distraction can be difficult for two reasons. One: The visual distraction alleviates their nervousness, anxiety, or stress around mealtimes. And two: It keeps them occupied and entertained. To take away both of those aspects at once can be challenging.

Some families like to cut out the distraction cold turkey. This means turning off the television and putting the iPad in another room immediately. Weaning all at once can be difficult but is much quicker. Typically, it leads to a tantrum (or several), but then children become accustomed to the new rules and begin to participate in mealtimes more thoroughly.

You could also make this transition more slowly. Typically, I recommend having your child make the transition from a screen, which is incredibly visually stimulating, to a book. The book is less visually stimulating than the screen but has many similar components. It's still something to look at and it still tells a story, but it isn't quite as visually distracting. Once they get accustomed to this, then you transition to a toy that's even less stimulating. This would be a toy that doesn't light up, make noise, or change during play. For example, wooden toys tend to be great for this. They're also easier to clean before and after mealtimes. A less distracting toy takes away the visually stimulating part of a book, but continues to provide the entertainment piece. A few days after this, you transition from allowing them to play with the wooden toy during meals to having the toy sit at the table and "watch" your child eat, though they're no longer allowed to play with it. This way they have something to look at if they need a visual distraction, but ultimately, the focus is on the meal. Last, you transition away from having a distraction at all, and the toy stays in their room. This method can take a bit longer than going cold turkey, but typically doesn't result in nearly so many tantrums. Both choices are wonderful, and what you choose will depend on what's best for your family. Whichever method you try, remember to be patient and persistent. You may find that your child has trouble letting go of the distraction at first, but if you keep at it, eventually, they'll come around.

Without visual distractions, your child will be primed to focus on their meal and to learn more adventurous eating habits!

5   Making Food Fun

Children of all ages learn best through play. Play is where children learn about their world, pick up new skills, and grow more confident. Knowing this, it makes sense that play is how they would become adventurous eaters too. There are lots of ways that we can make food and eating more fun.

The number one way that you can make food fun for your child is to enjoy it yourself. Show your children how to find the joy in cooking and baking, in taking in the scents of a new food, in sharing meals with others. Keep the focus on fun rather than on pressure or expectations. It's easy to stress about your child's getting enough nutrients, but your child can pick up on that stress, and it can make them stressed as well. By watching their parents have fun, play with food, and try new recipes and food combinations, your child will learn to find the joy in those things too.

We've all heard the phrase "Don't play with your food," but children actually need to do the opposite. Playing with their food will allow them to learn about it and get ready for the important steps of eating. Let them use food to build towers or to fight dragons. They can pretend their carrots are a car or their broccoli is a lion. You can have them pretend to be a dinosaur that only eats leafy greens, or a puppy eating its steak. Playing with their food will bring fun and joy to what may be a stressful experience right now.

In addition to setting up a low-stress, low-pressure environment for your child, there are lots of little things that you can do to make mealtime itself fun. Changing up the way that you serve their food can make their meal look more exciting. You can use cookie cutters to change the shape of their sandwiches, fruit, veggies, and more. Finding shapes that they like can increase their willingness to play pretend with it, can increase buy-in, and can give them something else to think about if they're nervous about the food itself. You could cut the food into the shape of a favorite character or animal. Have your child play pretend with the food-creature. They can explore the texture of the food by picking up the creature to have them walk, jump, or play. They can give their food-creature kisses and nibble on it too. Many of us loved eating animal crackers as kids. It's so fun to chomp away at different shapes, and we can expand that play and fun to all sorts of foods by using a cookie cutter.

You can also change around the presentation of your child's food by serving it with a toothpick or kebab stick rather than a utensil, or presenting it on a snack tray like hors d'oeuvres. Using a toothpick can help your child feel like a big kid and can add some variety to their eating experience. Much as serving appetizers on a nice tray can make them seem fancier and more special, creating fun experiences like this can help your child feel more daring in their eating. Some families find it helpful to make a snack tray full of healthy foods for those picky eaters who come home hungry from school. Rather than go to the cabinet for cookies and chips, they can go to their snack tray to find little bits of fruits, veggies, or proteins that they'd like to adventure with instead.

You can alternatively make mealtime fun by letting your child be a scientist in the kitchen. Let them help you try new recipes and experiment with what different mixtures taste like. They may not all taste amazing, but exploring and trying things out can add a spark of fun to your kitchen. When you and your child find a new recipe together, you can give them ownership over it by calling it "Trish's Vegetable Soup" or "Max's Fruit Salad." When your child has a recipe named after them, they'll be much more excited to try it and to share it with others.

In the era of social media, there are lots of ideas out there for how to creatively put your child's food on a plate. Organize their food into a rainbow or a happy face. Your child will have fun picking apart the picture and will be excited to try new foods if they're part of the image on the plate. You can even have your child participate in making pictures with their food. Hold a competition in your family for who can most creatively plate their food. Getting your whole family involved can increase your child's investment in their meal.

There are lots of fun ways to get your child involved in and excited about mealtime. Keep things light and playful and your child will follow suit. Remember to view play as learning and to give your child the chance to playfully explore their food.

Part Two

TACTILE

Your child's tactile system will probably teach them the most about food before they actually put it in their mouth. After they visually inspect food, they ascertain even more information—what texture the food is, how wet or dry it is, how hard it will be to chew, and so much more—through feeling it. This is why most babies like to play with their food and rub it around their plate (and hands, and face, and hair!).

As with all senses, every child has a different preference for what they like. We have preferences for the textures that we enjoy touching, are able to tolerate touching, and hate touching as adults too! For example, some people love kneading dough and find it incredibly relaxing, whereas others have a strong urge to wash their hands immediately afterward to cleanse themselves of that tactile sensation. As adults that are confident with new foods, we can use our other senses to tell us about what we're eating and then use utensils to bring it to our mouths. Kids have less experience extrapolating information about food and often rely on their sense of touch to learn more details about new foods. When children's tactile systems make them avoid new textures, it can cause problems.

In general, our tactile systems are most comfortable with dry, consistent textures, and less comfortable with things that are wet or gooey. For example, most everyone is comfortable touching a dry, plastic utensil, right? But how many people do you know would enjoy plunging their hands into a large bowl of jello? Far fewer, right? Many children see these preferences play out in their mealtime experiences as well. Children who are sensitive to tactile input may gravitate toward foods that are dry and consistent, like crackers and chips, and avoid foods that are wetter or have less predictable textures, like oranges or kiwis.

To see if your child's tactile system could be affecting their eating habits, try looking back to your list of the foods that they eat and their corresponding textures. Do you see a pattern? Do most or all of the foods that your child enjoys have a similar texture profile? If so, their tactile system could be a factor in their eating habits.

So what happens if they're sensitive to these different textures and don't like the feeling of some foods? This can often lead to children's being unwilling to bring that food to their mouth. As a general rule of thumb, children typically only feel comfortable eating things that they're comfortable touching.

With continued positive experiences with new textures, your child can actually develop new texture preferences and learn to tolerate and enjoy a wider variety of textures and foods. If your child is feeling unsure about a texture, you can help empower them by setting a good example. If you're not worried about mess, they won't be either. You can provide a towel for them to wipe off their own fingers, that way they can feel like they have an "escape plan" to get away from the texture if needed. You can also provide smaller bites so that it's a smaller (and therefore easier) amount of food to manage. For many children, a large bite of a new texture can feel overwhelming, but a small bite can be manageable.

Exploring your tactile sense doesn't need to be limited to the dining room either. You can have your child help with gardening or picking out ripe fruit at the grocery store. They can help mix while you're cooking or help knead together dough to make cookies. There are lots of ways for your child to explore their feeling sense. Lean into the mess and show your child how to have fun with it as well.

6   The Importance of Messy Eating

Polite manners indicate that you should never play with your food, but for our developing babies and toddlers, messy eating and playing with their food are some of the best things that your child can do to support their feeding development. Although we've all felt that urge to clean our babies' hands and face while they're eating, we don't want our children to miss out on all the learning opportunities that messy eating provides. As a busy parent, it can be hard to create a time and space for your child to make a mess. That being said, finding times for your child to explore their food will do much to help them become more adventurous and confident eaters.

Messy eating is your child's first opportunity for tactile-based sensory play. Messy eating gives your child a chance to explore and learn about their tactile sense in a safe way, with textures that can (and should!) go in their mouths. Messy play fosters creativity and imagination. Starting messy play young (as soon as they can sit independently) is the best way for your child to learn about and taste foods, and it gives them a chance to enhance their play skills.

At this age, every toy goes in their mouth. If food is the toy, it will eventually go in their mouth too, allowing them the chance to explore new tastes and textures in a fun, low pressure way. If your child is a little bit older and has never done messy food play, there are tons of benefits to starting at any age. It's never too late to let your child make a mess with their food.

Children often go through a number of stages of comfort with a new food before they're willing to eat it. Typically, one of the first steps is looking at a food, allowing it on their plate, or smelling it. Then they might touch it with their hands, lips, or tongue before actually taking a bite. If your child isn't touching their food, then they're skipping one of the first steps of trying a new food. If they never get to touch the food and get messy with it, they may have a difficult time moving onto those later steps of actually tasting and eating the food. Giving a child opportunities to touch new foods allows them to get comfortable with that food before bringing it to their mouth.

As adults, we can look at a food and make a pretty good guess about what that food will feel like in our mouths based on the appearance. We've had a lifetime of experience in looking at and trying foods, so we have a good mental catalog of foods and their textures. If the food looks hard, we'll probably have to chew with a lot of pressure to be able to safely swallow the food. If it looks similar to a fruit or vegetable, we can guess that it might have some juice inside it that we will feel in our mouths during chewing. Babies and toddlers have had limited opportunities to build ideas about food, as they haven't been alive long enough to have had those experiences or to have formed that mental catalog. They don't have the experience to be able to look at a food and decide how they'll need to manage that food in their mouth. They use their hands to explore those foods and to make those determinations for themselves (before they ever put it in their mouths!). A child might not know that a carrot is going to feel hard just by looking at it, but once they pick it up and bang it against their table or tray, they'll feel how hard it is. They may not know that an orange slice will be juicy just by looking at it, but when they squish it between their fingers, they'll realize just how juicy it is. After a chance to play with their food, they won't be surprised by the texture once it enters their mouth. Playing with their food gives them the knowledge they need to feel ready to take a bite.

Messy play with food helps your child learn about their body and increases their body awareness. In playing with their food and bringing it to their mouth, your child will learn:

- About their mouth, their teeth, their tongue, and their lips

- How food feels on each of those parts on their jaw, tongue, and lips, and how to move each of those parts together to eat

- How much pressure it takes to bring food to their mouth, and how far they need to open their mouth to get the food in

- How to get food off their lips and how to use their hands together to bring food to their face

There's so much for your child to learn about their own body, and messy play gives them a chance to do just that. It'll also allow their brains to learn about how to use their sensory systems and their movement systems together and how to integrate all that information at once.

Although messy play can be inconvenient, it's so important for eating and overall development. If the idea of a mess freaks you out, know that there are steps you can take to make messy play a little cleaner:

- Use a placemat or towel, even under their chair.

- Do mealtimes on easy surfaces, like hardwood or tile.

- Have a dedicated set of "messy play" clothes.

It's important to create an environment where you, as the parent, feel comfortable. If you're stressing about messy play, your child will too. Children learn best through play, so create a space and time where you feel comfortable and playful. Before you know it, your child will feel that way too.

Remember—developing confidence with foods takes time. One messy eating experience won't be enough for your child to immediately feel confident and adventurous with a new food. Messy play is something that needs to be integrated into their routine. To make this easier to fit into your routine consider:

- Planning messy play on bath days

- Eating outside

- Letting your child help you cook

Finally, keep in mind that messy food play doesn't have to happen at meals. You can schedule some messy food time when it's convenient for you, even if that's not at breakfast, lunch, or dinnertime. Mealtimes can be rushed and busy, so it's okay to sometimes schedule that messy play for other times of the day.

As I've shared, research shows that it can take up to forty exposures to a new food before a child will feel ready to try it, so if you're not initially successful, don't give up hope. Consistency is key to developing confidence with new foods. So pull out your phone for some cute, messy photos, and have fun with it!

7 Managing Tactile Defensiveness at the Dining Table

When you've noticed that your child is uncomfortable with touching new foods but want to encourage tactile sensory experiences, there are many steps you can take to make them more comfortable. Two of the main ways to help your child be more comfortable are to empower them and to role model for them.

To empower your child around their tactile system, it's important to help them feel like they can take care of and adjust for their sensory preferences independently. As adults, knowing how to extract ourselves from uncomfortable situations easily, quickly, and independently gives us confidence to try new, unknown experiences.

The same is true for children exploring new textures. If they feel like they need to wait for help to clean their hands of whatever offending texture is on them, then they'll be less likely to want to touch that texture in the first place. After all, who wants to sit in an uncomfortable position for several minutes while they wait for mom or dad to get a damp washcloth, come over, and wipe their hands? No child that I know! Instead, we want to prepare them to be able to wipe their own hands and faces so that they can feel confident in the knowledge that they can introduce themselves to new food textures without feeling overwhelmed.

To set your child up for success, you can provide two washcloths: one wet and one dry. Ensuring that the washcloths are there when they start their meal will save you from getting them once their hands are already messy and they're already feeling uncomfortable or uncertain. Then teach your child how to wipe their hands and face and encourage them to do it independently.

This can feel a little easier said than done though. In the moment, when your child has messy hands and feels overwhelmed, their brain isn't in a good state to learn. Instead, they may feel panicked or highly distracted with only one thought on the mind: *Get this off of me!* If you find yourself in this position, I suggest practicing hand washing separately from mealtimes first.

Many children like to have mom or dad clean them during mealtimes because your presence is soothing. Parents are one of children's most common coping strategies. Whenever they're hurt, or in pain, or uncomfortable, you're there to make things better, which is amazing. There are a million things to do during mealtimes, though, which means that you can't always be *right there.* You can slowly decrease the amount of help that you give them by saying, "You try wiping your hands first. I'll be there in a second to help get the rest of it." This gives them a chance to try being independent but with the safety net of knowing you'll be there to help, too. Eventually, you'll be able to fade back entirely.

Once your child is confidently wiping their hands themselves, you can model how you handle messes on your hands or face. You can comment if you get some food on your fingers or face and narrate how you're going to wipe it off in a calm manner. Showing your child that you're feeling confident with the mess will allow them to feel confident as well.

The flip side of this is that you don't want to hover over your child and their messes. Rather, try to let your child process them on their own. For example, if you see food on your child's forehead, you may feel the urge to immediately wipe it off or to encourage them to wipe it off themselves before it gets in their hair. You'll want to try to refrain from doing that as much as possible, no matter how painful it is to watch that mess. When you interrupt a meal to clean them, you're sending the message that cleanliness is the most important thing. This reinforces their worries about that mess and puts their tactile system into high alert. Suddenly, their tactile system is constantly watching out for any potential mess. For sensitive children, this is the last thing that we want. Rather, we want them to be able to feel comfortable with food textures and to relax with them.

Learning to eat will take some trial and error for your child, and that process will be messy. That's okay. Try to embrace that and show your child through your modeling and actions that you feel comfortable with mess, and that they can too. After all, there's plenty of time for cleanup once you're done eating!

8 Introducing Other Tactile Sensations

If your child is too uncomfortable with the sensation of mess on their fingers to even be willing to touch their food, you can try creating some playful experiences around other tactile sensations. The idea of touching uncomfortable textures might be easier if they're not food and the child doesn't have the inherent pressure and expectation to put them in their mouth.

Many people like to use "sensory bins," which are basically just a box full of fun things to feel. I've seen children enjoy dry beans, dry rice, sand, clay, pasta, shredded paper, salt, water beads, and more. You can put pretty much anything in there and have a blast with it. As with foods, dry textures are easier to touch than wet ones, so keep that in mind while choosing play activities with your child.

If your child doesn't want to touch the objects in your sensory bin, you can always ease your child into touching them by giving them tongs or utensils to touch it with first. Putting toy figurines in the bin to set the scene or hiding puzzle pieces in the bin's contents can be engaging and exciting ways to get them involved.

You can also take your play out to nature and work together to gather objects with all sorts of tactile profiles. Gather sticks, leaves, dirt, sand, and grass to make your own craft. All of these objects can help your child become more comfortable with touching new and different textures.

Once your child has become comfortable with touching a variety of nonfood textures, you can transition back to food items. As an intermediary step, start by creating tactile learning experiences outside of mealtimes. Cooking together can be a great example of this. Your child can start to learn about the textures of foods before there's the direct pressure to eat it.

You could also go to places outside the house for these learning experiences. Places like farmer's markets, grocery stores, and berry patches are excellent places to gain exposure to food textures before they're on your plate. Then you can have the added benefit of bringing those foods home for cooking and dinner!

9   Introducing New Food Textures

I always think back to those Halloween grab bags at parties and carnivals, where you have to stick your hand in a hidden bag, feel what's inside, and guess what it is. Sometimes you'd find grapes, and they would say that it was eyeballs, or cooked pasta, and they'd pretend it was guts. That experience was pretty nerve racking for most people involved. Not knowing what to expect can be scary. Most people would feel comfortable picking up grapes if they could see them, but when they're in a hidden bag, many people visibly recoil. The same can be said for children in trying and touching new foods.

When you want to introduce your child to new food textures, start with thinking about what textures they're most comfortable with. Do they prefer wet foods, like juicy fruits, or dry foods, like toast? Once you know their preferences, it's much easier to think about the next steps.

To learn more about their preferences, consider answering the following questions, either on a piece of paper or on the worksheet listed on New Harbinger's website for this book at http://www.newharbinger.com/49524:

- What are your child's favorite foods?

- Is this food's texture dry or wet?

- Is it crunchy or chewy?

- If you hold it in your mouth for a few seconds, what does it feel like?

- Is the texture the same throughout or does it change as you chew it?

- Does the food involve one texture (like cheese) or multiple textures (like pizza, which has cheese, bread, sauce, and possibly toppings too)?

Now that you have your list, what patterns do you see? Do they have favorite categories of textures? If they do, that's what you'll want to use for your starting point.

When introducing new food textures, you always want to start slowly. There are two paths that you can take to introduce your child to new foods: slowly changing their preferred texture to a new texture, or combining their preferred texture with a new texture, like a dip.

Many children with texture preferences tend to prefer dry, crunchy textures, like crackers. They enjoy these because they're dry, not sticky, and have consistent texture throughout. When you bite a blueberry, it could be very juicy or less juicy, and you don't always know what you're going to get texture-wise. With crackers, the texture is always the same.

If your child enjoys crackers and you want to branch into some new textures, you could try slowly changing the texture. When you make those little changes, you want to start by thinking about foods that are similar to the food that they like. For example, very crispy toast is very similar to crackers. Once they learn to feel confident with crispy toast, you could slowly toast the bread less and less until they're eating fresh bread, which is soft and squishy. To change the texture even more, you could move from fresh bread to rolls, or to different types of bread. White bread and wheat bread have very different textures. If you want to use bread to introduce your child to wetter textures, you could make a bread pudding or French toast.

Another way that you can introduce your child to new textures is to try combining preferred and non-preferred textures. An example of this would be using a dip. When you combine two textures, you want to start with a large amount of the preferred food and a tiny amount of the new texture. If you wanted to use a cracker to introduce a new, wetter texture food (like peanut butter), you would want to start with a whole cracker and the tiniest dab of peanut butter that you can put on. Initially, the peanut butter may cover only 1 percent of the cracker, and that's totally okay. This allows you to make that transition slowly and then eventually work up to changing the texture further.

Once your child is comfortable with a small amount of peanut butter, you can slowly increase it until the entire cracker is covered. Once they're feeling confident with peanut butter crackers, you could modify the texture even further by combining it with a little bit of jelly, again slowly working your way up to more. Eventually, your child will feel comfortable with the texture of a peanut butter and jelly cracker sandwich, which has three separate and very different textures in it.

Depending on the child, this transition can happen quickly, like in the span of one meal, or over a longer period of time, like several weeks or months. It all depends on how your child's body processes that change and what their confidence level is with new things. Over time, these introductions will get quicker and quicker.

You can make these slow texture introductions with any food. In this chapter, I gave the example of starting with crackers and working your way toward sandwiches, but you can make these transitions with anything. The important parts to remember are to make slow changes over time and to branch between familiar foods and similar, less familiar foods.

I like to make a diagram where I start with a favorite food and draw branches out for similar foods that I want to help them learn to love. For this cracker example, it might look something like this:

Toast   fresh bread   French toast

Crackers

Cracker with   Cracker with peanut butter
peanut butter   and jelly

As you're introducing your child to new foods, talk about textures with them. You can talk about the textures of both food and non-food items. Teach them different adjectives that they can use to describe textures. Is it bumpy, smooth, slimy, dry, sticky, crumbly, or wet? There are so many words that can describe foods, and knowing what a food is going to feel like before they feel it (or eat it) will help them feel more confident. Empowering them with a more robust vocabulary around food textures will help them know what to expect and prepare their bodies for the tactile sensation.

By giving your child the tools they need, and by introducing new textures with little steps, they'll feel more confident branching to new textures and expanding their list of preferred foods beyond their favorite food texture.

Part Three

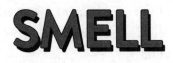

SMELL

Smell is such an exciting sense because it's intimately connected with our sense of taste. Specialized cells in our noses pick up airborne odor molecules from food, and those cells send a signal to our brain about what we're smelling. Our senses of smell and taste mix together at the back of our throat and combine to interpret whatever food we're eating. Because of this, our sense of smell is a very important factor in eating, trying new foods, fighting picky eating.

Some people never seem to pick up on new scents, while others notice every tiny smell. A smell that may be hardly noticeable to you may be overwhelming to your child.

Children who prefer very strong-smelling foods can be bored or understimulated by bland foods. For these children, many recipes can be easily modified with additional spices or sauces.

Children who are sensitive to new or strong smells are particularly vulnerable to becoming picky eaters because they tend to avoid strong-smelling foods. After all, if the smell of a food makes you gag, why would you put it in your mouth? Evolution taught your child to stay away from foods that smell bad to them because those foods could be dangerous. Unfortunately, that pattern doesn't always work the way it should and often leads children to avoid safe foods, particularly when their sensory processing of smell isn't working optimally. It can even turn into a cyclical pattern. When a food's smell upsets your child's nervous system, they're more likely to avoid that food. When they avoid a perceived negative food smell, they reinforce this pattern and can become more sensitive. The cycle can also work in the reverse direction: extremely picky eaters often avoid so many smells that they limit their olfactory system's exposure (the sensory system used for smelling), and through this avoidance, they can become more sensitive.

All this means that the key to making your child more comfortable with new smells is to help them have more positive experiences with smells. Of course, you don't want to overwhelm them and make them miserable, but rather find fun ways to push the envelope and help them get more comfortable with new smells.

Read on in this section for more ways to strengthen their smell processing and to adjust their mealtime routine for more adventurous eating.

10 Adjusting the Environment

Have you ever made the most fabulous dinner only to have your child show up to the table and gag at the smell? How frustrating is that? It's important to remember that this isn't something they can control and certainly isn't a commentary on your cooking! Their nervous system is just learning to process and modulate their response to olfactory input. It's important to take this sensitivity seriously but not personally. As with all your child's traits that make them wonderful and unique, it's not your fault. Luckily though, there are many things you can do to make mealtimes easier.

Being compassionate about your child's olfactory preferences doesn't mean avoiding all the smells they dislike. In fact, it can mean the opposite. Giving your child positive olfactory experiences will help them learn to tolerate and enjoy more smells and will help them to find mealtimes more enjoyable.

A cool thing about our sense of smell is that it adjusts quickly. After all, how often have you walked into your favorite restaurant and felt overcome by how good it smells, only to stop noticing the smell before your order even arrives? We can take advantage of this to help your child become less overwhelmed by the smell of food.

You can start adjusting the environment before you even sit down to eat. Try having your child come help or "supervise" your cooking in the kitchen. They can do homework nearby or help you gather the ingredients. Before you start cooking, your kitchen probably doesn't smell like much, and your child probably feels very comfortable in there. The smell will slowly start building as you cook. By the time you're done cooking, and once all the ingredients have been combined, the smell will have spread throughout the kitchen and will be at its strongest. If your child is present at the start of your cooking, their body will have a chance to acclimate to the smell as it builds. Of course, this isn't always possible with evening routines but is definitely worthwhile when you can manage it. If you can't have them there to help you with cooking, at least give them a warning that you're going to start cooking. They'll start to regulate their bodies and prepare for the upcoming olfactory experience. By avoiding the surprise, you can limit gagging episodes.

Once you start the meal, you'll want to make the environment as calm as possible. This will mean not reacting if your child gags (or even vomits) from the smell. Keeping a straight face can feel nearly impossible. After all, it's natural instinct to want to run to their aid and to make a fuss over them and make sure they're okay. This can actually make it worse though. Gagging can be a little scary for them too, and if you make a big show of supporting them, then it reinforces the idea that something is very wrong. If you stay calm and act like everything's fine, they'll believe that too.

We often talk about how children can coregulate, which means their body can adjust toward the energy of the people around them. Have you ever been around a nervous person who makes you nervous too? Or have you ever met someone that seems to radiate calm energy and always make you feel warm and safe, no matter what's going on? You want to be that second person for your child. If you stay calm and minimally react to their gagging, you'll send the message that everything is okay. This will calm their nervous system and help them relax and acclimate to the smell. It will also help subdue their instinct to avoid the food that they consider danger-ous because of gagging.

To get through a mealtime, you can minimize the power of the smell, like move the food further away from your child. Sometimes compassion-ately moving the food further down the table, relocating it into the kitchen, or covering it with a lid can help limit the strength of the smell without allowing your child to avoid the smell altogether. You could open a window or turn a fan on. It may not be enough, and the weather may not allow for it all year long, but having some fresh air could go a long way toward ven-tilating a room and helping your child stay more engaged with the meal.

Beyond changing the setup of the room and table, you could give them some compensatory strategies to get through the meal comfortably. Many children enjoy using a familiar scent on a band or scrunchie that they wear on their wrist. When they're feeling overwhelmed, they can bring their wrist to their nose to override the noxious smell. Allow your child to choose a scent for themselves so it's one that they're comfortable with. The last thing they want is to have one overwhelming smell on their dinner plate and another on their wrist.

It can also be helpful to provide them with a napkin or handkerchief that they can use to block their nose for the first part of the meal. Although it's not the best table manners, it can help them get through the first part of the meal until their body adjusts and the scent becomes slightly less overpowering.

Regardless of how their olfactory process is working for them at that moment, there are many things that you can do to help give your child the confidence to participate in a meal. Being present and participatory in mealtimes—making mealtimes mindful experiences in which everyone's engaged, getting kids involved in meal preparation and cleanup as well as eating, and other such strategies—can decrease picky eating. The next chapter will dive more into how to desensitize their olfactory processing so that they rely on these compensatory strategies less and less as time goes on.

11 Helping Your Child with New Smells

If your child is sensitive to smell, it can be hard to accommodate their preferences, since smells are everywhere and they travel so easily. It's not easy to limit the smell of dinner in the oven as it spreads through the house. Luckily, this also means that smell is a very commonly activated sense in our day-to-day lives, and there are many opportunities in your normal routine to help strengthen their smell processing.

For a child that's sensitive to smells, you'll want to expose them to a variety of new smells in a positive and non-overwhelming way. Starting small and keeping these experiences enjoyable will build confidence and help desensitize them to more food scents later on. It can teach their brain how to more effectively process this olfactory input and to modulate the nervous system's reaction to it so that they no longer feel uncomfortable around scents, gag, or vomit.

Support your child's exploration of their sense of smell by creating opportunities for them to interact with different smells in their day-to-day life. Take a walk through the candle or produce aisles at the grocery store and sample different smells. Explore the garden or farmer's market and compare smells between different forms of produce or flowers.

Cooking food together is a huge opportunity for teaching their body how to better process smells. While cooking, smells tend to build throughout the cooking process. This gives your child's body a chance to adjust to the smells throughout the process rather than be exposed to the stronger smell at the end of the meal.

Cooking together is a beautiful opportunity for you to teach your child about ingredients and what they smell like. You can go through your spice cabinet and take turns smelling the spices and deciding what to add. When your child can smell the ingredients separately before adding them together, it empowers them to feel more confident mixing flavors and helps their body prepare for the combination of smells before they're mixed.

It can be fun to involve new smells in play activities. You can add olfactory input into many of their favorite games. For example, if they love playing with play dough, try adding a small scent or some dried spices, like lavender, into it. Scented doughs can be a blast to play with, and the dough gives them something else to focus on while their body is working on processing the olfactory input.

Many families like to make sensory bins, if those are something that your child enjoys playing with. If your child has a favorite sensory bin, you can easily modify it to stimulate their olfactory sense as well. Some families like to include dried flowers or dried whole spices, like cinnamon sticks, into them. Others include essential oils for a fun, scented experience. With these, remember that a little goes a long way! When you're sprinkling an essential oil over a large bin of rice, it really only needs a drop or two.

You can make scented spray bottles with water and spices or other scents and involve these in their play. Maybe the mist from the spray bottle is a perfume for their favorite train toy, or it could be a rare scented rain that their toy figurine has to solve the mystery of. With creativity, the sky is the limit on ways to incorporate scent into their play.

Many stores make a variety of scented toys and art supplies. There are scented markers, stamps, crayons, and more! The nice thing about scented writing implements is that they often come with a cap or some sort of carrying case. If your child begins to feel overwhelmed by the scent, they can always close the cap or put away the implement into its storage case.

With all of these desensitization experiences, make sure to keep them very fun and enjoyable. The goal is never to make your child uncomfortable or unhappy. Rather, it's to give their body and brain little challenges they can easily complete so that they can slowly build their skills in processing olfactory input.

I recommend keeping all these activities to a short time limit as you start out. You can always build as they feel more comfortable and confident in handling those smells. And if, in any of these experiences, you find that your child is feeling uncomfortable or overwhelmed, it's good to take a short step away from the activity. After all, we want to keep these experiences enjoyable and end them while they're still having fun. This will leave them raring to go for the next time!

With more and more opportunities to practice tolerating new smells, your child will feel more confident with handling them in all areas of life (including at the dining table!).

12　Building a Smell Vocabulary

Children often don't have the words to talk about sensitivities to smell. Instead, their body has a huge reaction to the scent, and they feel uncomfortable. This discomfort contributes to their needing to avoid that scent (and talking about it) as much as possible.

One thing that we know about avoidance is it can ultimately make our body's reaction to discomfort worse. Avoiding something reinforces the neurological pathway in our brain that says, "This is something dangerous that we need to avoid." This reinforcement can happen very frequently with children that are uncomfortable or gag with strong scents. The scent causes their body to have a strong adverse reaction, so they think, *I need to avoid this at all costs.* Avoiding the scent then makes their body even more sensitive to those types of input, making the reaction even worse the next time it happens.

Helping your child build a vocabulary to talk about scents, especially ones that they find noxious, can help empower them to better handle it. Having words that they can put to their feelings and experiences can give them so much more confidence. It allows them to track patterns in their own body, prepare for the way it might react, and advocate for their own needs.

A strong vocabulary for scents also allows them to better prepare for different types of olfactory input. If someone tries to warn you that a restaurant smells "garlicky," but you don't know what the word garlicky means, the scent of garlic could be surprising and shocking. However, if this sounds familiar, then you can prepare your body and enter the restaurant with more confidence.

Giving your child a wide vocabulary of descriptive words for scents will help them prepare for and control their body's reaction to olfactory input more successfully. Try talking about how things smell in the course of your day-to-day life. When you notice smells, talk about and label them.

I strongly advise sticking to neutral words as much as you can. If you label something as "nasty" or "great," it encourages your child to think it a dichotomy where everything is black or white, and all smells are good or bad. The problem with polarization is that a smell-sensitive child might label 99 percent of smells as "bad." This thought pattern reinforces the body's response that it really is bad. In contrast if you think of smells on a scale of 1–10, with one being noxious and ten being most favorable, most smells will fall somewhere in the middle for most of us. By using more descriptive and neutral words, you help your child develop a vocabulary to reflect this phenomenon and a vocabulary to reinforce the idea that their body can tolerate and enjoy a wider variety of scents. Framing different olfactory experiences like this can also reinforce the idea that even non-preferred smells can be worth investigating and learning about, helping your child feel confident in exploring new food experiences rather than shut down.

It can further be helpful to talk to your child about "big smells" versus "small smells." A big smell is something that smells really strong, whereas a food with a small smell might be hardly noticeable. Something that is a big smell for your child may be a small or medium smell for you, and vice versa. Giving your child the language around big and small smells will likewise help them prepare for and describe their body's reaction around their olfactory sense. Over time they'll be able to see how something that might have been a huge, gigantic, overwhelming smell turns into a medium or tolerable smell with practice and continued exposure.

Talk about different smells both away from and at the dining table. Having words to use to think about the smell of foods—like fruity, earthy, floral, or fresh—will help your child think about and feel more comfortable using their sense of smell to explore their foods. Try encouraging your child to smell their foods before eating them and to put a label to them. This helps children start to build a flavor profile and get ready for trying new foods, and it also provides a fun, low-pressure way for them to playfully get comfortable with smells.

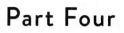

Part Four

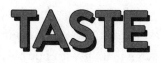

TASTE

Taste is probably the most intuitive sense when it comes to eating. After all, we do put the food in our mouths to taste and eat it! There's a lot to know and understand about your child's sense of taste though, so that you can best support them in expanding their taste preferences.

When food reaches our tongue, the food interacts with taste receptor cells that are located on our taste buds. These taste receptors communicate to our brain what they think the food tastes like.

Our bodies are equipped to identify five basic types of taste: sweet, sour, salty, bitter, and savory (also known as umami). Spicy foods can also instigate a reaction (in combination with our taste perception) that activates our nerves to communicate the heat of that particular food. Similarly, our bodies can perceive "cool" foods, like ones with minty flavor.

The way that our bodies react to each of these types of taste can vary though. We see that in the fact that everyone has different tastes. One person's favorite food might be another person's least favorite. This preference for taste starts to develop very early in life—in utero! (Nehring et al. 2015) What pregnant mothers eat can affect the taste of their amniotic fluid, which babies start to swallow around twelve weeks after conception. Babies develop preferences through exposures to what their mother eats during pregnancy and then during breastfeeding (if she chooses to do so). These early exposures can be valuable, but later experiences through childhood and beyond are just as important.

The great news about preferences is that everyone can learn to like every type of food. It just takes skillful repetition! Studies show that it takes about twenty separate times of trying a food before you learn to like it (Carruth and Skinner 2000). This can feel like forever, right? But this section will guide you through some ways to speed this up and make the most of your child's food experiences to help expand their palate.

13 Food Chaining

Food chaining was developed by Cheri Fraker, a speech therapist and feeding therapist, and is the process of introducing your child to new foods that are similar to foods that they already like. That is, rather than introduce a picky eater to all sorts of different foods at once, you introduce them to foods that are similar to ones that are familiar and comfortable for them (Fraker et al. 2007).

For example, if your child really loves chicken nuggets, food chaining would suggest that they might like fish sticks, fried mozzarella sticks, or breaded cauliflower nuggets. All three of these foods have similar appearances (breaded), similar textures (crunchy on the outside and soft in the inside), and taste (fried). Because they look and taste similar to chicken nuggets, a chicken nugget lover would be more likely to explore and enjoy these foods than they would something completely different, like a raw carrot.

With food chaining, anything can link two foods together. In making a food chain, we want to start with a food that they're comfortable with and modify it slightly so that, over time and with numerous modifications, we end up at a new food.

One thing to keep in mind with forming bridges is that we only want to change one sense's perception at a time. If we change what the food tastes like, we want to keep the appearance, smell, texture, and any auditory input that they get while chewing as similar as possible. One example of this would be transitioning from pink-colored vanilla yogurt to strawberry yogurt. The yogurt remains the same color, smell, texture, and auditory input, but our taste perception of it changes. The similarities between strawberry yogurt and pink-colored vanilla yogurt help the child feel more confident and make the jump to a new flavor of yogurt. From there they could branch to strawberry yogurt with chunks of strawberries in it, eventually to fresh whole strawberries.

Depending on how particular your child is, these steps may need to be larger or smaller than those two examples. Some children require lots of modifications, with lots of time between new modifications. For instance, a very picky child that accepts a small number of foods may only feel comfortable with smaller steps between familiar and new foods. Let's return to the example of chicken nuggets. In this example, let's consider a child who only enjoys one specific brand of chicken nuggets and won't eat any other meats. With a child with rigid expectations like this, we may start by trying new brands of the same shape of chicken nuggets, so it has a slightly different flavor but all our other sensory experiences remain the same. Then we could move on to chicken nuggets that have a different shape, so the taste remains the same but the visual appearance changes. Only once they were comfortable with these little varieties would we move on to fish sticks or the other examples noted above. Chaining in this way can take some time, but the results are worth it. Slowly but surely, your child will expand their food preferences, one step (or link) at a time.

When making these changes, I recommend not lying to your child about changing their food. That being said, you don't want to draw specific attention to the changes either. For example, when serving a new brand of chicken nuggets, you could tell your child, "We're having chicken nuggets for dinner." If they notice it's not what they're used to, it's okay to confirm, "Yes, this is a different type of chicken nugget. It's still chicken nuggets though." This could be an opportunity to talk about similarities between the new chicken nuggets and their familiar chicken nugget brand. You may want to stay away from highlighting differences yourself, but you can corroborate your child's observations.

Another way that you can help your child bridge from one food to another is through dips. Does your child have a favorite dip that they love to put on everything? Use that as a bridge! If you have a ketchup fan, provide ketchup as a side with new foods. Because the ketchup feels familiar, they'll feel more confident in trying that food, even if it's totally unfamiliar. Research shows that dips significantly increase children's vegetable and meat consumption (Nekitsing et al. 2018). Anything can be a dip. If your child likes yogurt or peanut butter, feel free to use that as a dip. When your child uses a dip, they may start by just licking the dip off their meat or veggies. In doing so, they'll start to get a taste for the food underneath. Eventually, they'll feel more comfortable eating pieces of it too.

When looking at food chaining with your child, you want to first meet your child where they are. If you try to push them too far, too fast, they'll feel overwhelmed and intimidated. Introducing children to new foods is always a marathon and not a sprint.

Start by taking a look at their preferences and make a list of new foods that you would like them to add to their repertoire. From there you can make a game plan for what steps they need to take to get from point A to point B. Consider foods that taste similar to foods that your child already likes.

Even if the new foods that your child learns to enjoy are very similar to foods that they're already eating, any new food still adds variety to their nutritional intake and confidence to their approach to eating! And before you know it, little chains add up to big steps!

14　Preventing Food Jags

First, you're probably wondering what a food jag is. Food jag is a name for when your child will only eat one food, or a very small group of foods, for meal after meal after meal.

It can be so frustrating, and stressful, when all your child wants for days on end is mac and cheese or chicken nuggets. Food jags can make mealtimes challenging and disrupt family routines; not to mention, you may worry if your child is getting all the nutrients they need. But how can we stop them from happening?

First, know that food jags are incredibly common for both toddlers and picky eaters. Being a toddler is all about learning that you can control your environment and testing out the boundaries of that control. At the end of the day, what can our toddlers really control? As parents, we dictate most of their day for them. We tell them when they're getting dressed, getting in the car, taking a nap, and so on. One thing that they can control is what goes in their mouth. This is why previously easy-to-feed babies can become picky eaters between eighteen months and two years old.

In addition to craving that control, toddlers love routine. And what's more routine than eating the same food for several meals in a row?

Lack of control is also why toddlers have so many tantrums. They're in a period of so much growth and so many new experiences, and while this is exciting, it can be stressful too. Practicing and learning healthy coping skills are good things to do in response; it can unfortunately take some time. Sometimes children fall back on food as a more immediate way to soothe themselves, the way they did as babies. Everyone has comfort foods, and children typically fall back on these during their food jags.

Regardless of why your child is having a food jag, it's important to parent them through this so that they can add more foods back into their diet at the end and not forget about them forever. And most kids on food jags, even picky eaters, will add the foods they cut out back into their routine diet eventually.

One of the biggest things to consider before and during a food jag is rotating foods. Picky eaters, by definition, tend to limit themselves to a small number of foods. And when a child is eating the same foods over and over, they become more prone to food jagging. What's more, in the middle of a jag, when they have had the same foods, with the same nutrients, day after day, their bodies sometimes send a message to the brain: "We don't need any more of this food! Stop eating it." So the child stops. And this can very easily and quickly spiral. If a picky eater only has five foods that they enjoy, and they eat all five of those foods every day, they may cut out one (or more) from their repertoire. Then they're down to even fewer foods, which they have to eat with more frequency to meet their caloric needs— putting them at even further risk of additional food jagging.

Rotating the foods your child eats can stop this cycle. Generally, we aim not to serve the same food two days in a row. For example, don't fall into the habit of serving the same fruit at every lunchtime meal. I recommend keeping a journal of what you're feeding your child to help ensure enough variety. Being a parent can be exhausting and stressful, and it's easy to fall into too consistent patterns. Varying your child's routine will help prevent your child from falling into a food jag and limiting themselves to just one familiar food.

If your child is very picky, this may be hard to do. Try finding little ways to vary their food. For example, if toast is one of the only foods that they'll accept, try making it slightly different each day. You could make it with different types of bread, or with different toppings. Any little change will make a big difference, and you can continue to chain those little changes into bigger ones, as I described in the previous chapter.

Because picky eating is often about wanting control, find ways to collaborate with your children so that they feel like active participants in their own feeding experiences. It can help to give two options that you're okay with so that your child practices independence and making a choice, and you're still in a position to make sure that they're getting the nutrients that they need.

For example, you could ask your child, "It's snack time. Would you like apples or carrots?" This way you offer foods that you're okay with, and they still feel like they're in control of their food intake. If your child is on a food jag and responds that they only want their preferred food (let's say mac and cheese), you could respond, "That's not a choice right now. We can have mac and cheese again tomorrow. Right now your choices are apples or carrots. Which would you like?" Then the following day, you can follow up with them: "Yesterday you said you wanted mac and cheese, and I said we could have it today. Would you still like that or would you like a cheese stick?" Offering choices takes a lot of the fight and stress out of mealtime options, and it stops you from being your child's short-order cook.

Sometimes though, we can't offer choices in what foods we're offering for a whole variety of reasons. That doesn't mean that you can't still offer choices though. You could offer, "Would you like the blue plate or the brown plate for snack today?" The key is to always make sure that you are okay with both the choices that you're offering.

If you have a really picky eater, you might be thinking, *I don't even have two food choices that my child might eat!* Even if your child only eats one food, there are still ways to integrate some variety. If your child is stuck on yogurt, for example, you could try different flavors, or using the yogurt as a dip instead of eating it out of a bowl. Or, if your child is stuck on chicken nuggets, you could get different shape chicken nuggets, serve them whole or cut up, or with a sauce. There are always ways to add variety that will help prevent your child from becoming too rigid in their eating routines. The changes in the food don't have to be huge to make a huge difference for your child.

That said, once you've set a choice or expectation, consistency is crucial. If you waffle or change your mind, then your child will feel like the choices that you offer are up for negotiation. Once that happens, it'll be significantly harder to get your child to make a choice that you're okay with, because they'll feel like if they just keep pushing, they might get you to change your mind again. Stay consistent. Your child will realize that the options you give aren't up for debate, and they'll be much more likely to participate in the mealtime that you've set up.

One way to help your child start to think about new foods can be to involve them in food preparation. Thinking about and interacting with their foods before mealtime will allow your child to start to increase their comfort with those foods and will give them a feeling of investment in the meal.

There are many ways to safely involve your child in meal prep at any age. Starting as a baby, they can come with you to the grocery store. You can talk about the foods that you see. That apple is red, this carrot is hard, that peach is fuzzy. This starts to give your child words for talking about new foods and gives them positive ways to think about them.

As they get older, they can help mix or pour, or can peek in the microwave or oven to watch their food cook. Being involved in the process will allow your child to feel proud about the meal that they've created and will start to give them an understanding of the texture of the food that they're going to eat. Understanding texture before eating is so important because it shows children how they'll need to chew once that food is in their mouth. If the food is something that they cannot safely help make, they could help put the food on their plate or could help clean up at the end. Many toddlers love to play pretend kitchen, and creating opportunities for them to be involved in cooking can make food seem fun and exciting. Involving your child with food prep at an early age can help prevent food jags, as they'll have a larger selection of familiar foods, feel more confident in handling those foods, and be more likely to eat them.

When you're looking at your child's feeding experience, you and your child share equal but separate responsibilities. As registered dietician and family therapist Ellyn Satter posits, parents are responsible for what, when, and where their child eats. The child is responsible for how much they actually eat (Satter 2000). Lots of parents complain about how their child's diet has too much junk food in it. But ultimately, that's your responsibility. Parents talk about how they're upset that their child snacks all day long. That's your responsibility. Parents talk about how it's frustrating that their child walks around with their food and leaves it all around the house. That's your responsibility.

To avoid unnecessary stress, focus on the things that you can control and not on the things you can't. If your child only tries one bite of what you offer, that's not something that you can control. You can only control what you offer. Let your child worry about how much they're going to eat, and you worry about what you're going to make available to them. Sharing responsibility like that helps take unnecessary stress and burden off both you and your child.

Sometimes parents worry that their child will be hungry if they don't eat what's offered, and want to offer a preferred food immediately after. If your child feels like they have the option to wait it out and get a preferred food afterward, they're going to choose to do that. If your child has difficulty growing and your pediatrician has concerns about their growth, you may have to adjust their mealtime routine. For typically developing and growing children however, skipping one snack or meal will not disrupt their growth. They'll make up those calories later on in the day.

Lots of children like to refuse food at mealtimes and then, immediately after the dishes are cleared, come up to you and say, "I'm hungry! Can I have a snack?" An easy way to address this situation is to save your child's unfinished portion of their meal in the fridge. Then, when they come up to you later in the evening, you can reoffer it to them (provided it's a food that won't spoil). If they're really hungry, they'll eat it. If not, try to take that burden off yourself and allow them to be responsible for how much they eat.

Part of a food jag is about your child's trying to create routine for themselves. If they eat the same food at every meal, life feels more consistent and predictable. As a parent, your role in supporting them through this is to create routine in both food-related and non-food-related aspects of their lives. Children thrive in routine.

Promoting routines will help your child feel safer and more willing to adventure at the dining table. Maintain consistent wake-up, bed, and nap times. Try to keep consistent meal and snack times. Real life can be messy, difficult, and hard to predict. Anything that you can do to make it feel more predictable for your child will help. If your schedule varies, you could talk to your child about what your day is going to look like. For example, "After we get dressed, we're going to go to the library," or, "I know we had talked about going to the park today, but it's too rainy. Instead, we could read a book or color." Telling your child what to predict, or offering choices in routine, can help them feel like life is more predictable. When their routine is predictable, they'll feel more secure and more ready to branch out when it comes to their eating.

At the end of the day, don't stress. Food jags happen for many children. While it can be easy to put a lot of stress on ourselves as parents, it's important to stay relaxed around mealtimes. When you're stressed, your child is going to pick up on that, and it can cause anxiety for them as well. Two weeks of a limited diet here and there aren't going to cause a huge nutritional deficit for your child. Stay relaxed and provide lots of opportunities for your child to try new foods, and your adventurous eater will be back before you know it.

15 Empowering Children and Developing Their Tastes

There are many ways to empower your child. One of the most powerful things that you can do for your child is to model how to try new foods with curiosity rather than judgment. Being a good model looks like demonstrating all the mealtime behaviors that you want your child to have as well. If you want your child to remain seated at the table during mealtimes but you are constantly running back into the kitchen, it sends mixed messages about your expectations for your child. By staying at the table and engaging positively with all foods, preferred and non-preferred alike, you'll encourage the behaviors that you want to see.

As a parent, you are your child's number one role model. They look up to you for everything, including what and how to eat. If you model trying new foods, your child will think that looks fun and want to try as well.

In being a good mealtime role model, you can use your actions to show your child how to be open minded with your own non-preferred foods. Your child learns by copying you. If you say, "I don't like that!" then your child will learn to say that too. Instead, you could show them how to be brave about trying something by saying, "I'm not so sure about this, yet. What could we do to make it taste better?" Emphasizing that you don't like it yet implies that there are other things that you can do to learn to like or modify the food so that you enjoy it more. And this is absolutely true! So many foods are an acquired taste or are better enjoyed with some extra seasoning or other modifications. There are ways for all people to enjoy all foods—it can just take some time, patience, and exposure. So, you can guide your child through ways to modify the taste of something, like seasonings or sauces. Help your child move from feeling apprehensive about new tastes to finding fun in the adventure.

Talking about this with your child shows your child that it's okay not to like every food right off the bat, but that you shouldn't give up on it. It just means that you have more to explore before you find a way that you love it. And there's something to appreciate even in the act of trying foods you hate. In doing this, you'll reinforce the principle that approaching foods (that you may otherwise avoid) with curiosity and determination before you judge them is, in and of itself, valuable.

When setting the table for dinner, you can try serving food family style. This way your child has an opportunity to look at and inspect the food without any pressure to eat it. You can have everyone in your family take turns serving the food to others. This way, they use a spoon to dig through the food and start to experience its texture even before they try it.

In addition to modeling curiosity and eating family style, we want to find ways to frame these experiences in a positive way, which will set our children up for success in trying new foods. When our brain pairs positive messages with memories of past challenges, these optimistic thoughts can powerfully affect our openness to adventures of all kinds. For example, when recalling learning to ride a bike, we might remember, *I fell but I got back up and tried again until I got it.* Then when we face a new physical challenge, we can remind ourselves that while yes, this is hard, we have done and can do hard things.

We want to give our children positive phrases to use around eating too. We can assist our children in creating their own food narrative: *Once I had to try chicken nuggets for the first time and now they're my favorite food. Maybe my next new food will be my new favorite.* Having positive messages and affirmations in their head can help eliminate negative thoughts, like *I won't like it* or *This will be gross.* It can also build your child's confidence and their image of themselves as an adventurous eater.

It can also help your child to use neutral words to describe their food. Some picky eaters end up categorizing foods into "good" or "bad." They see these foods in black and white. Foods are favorites or disgusting, with no middle ground. In reality, as adults the majority of foods that we eat fall somewhere in that gray area. We all have favorite foods, but we also have foods that we eat because they're okay, they're convenient, someone pre-pared them for us, or any other reason. We eat lots of foods beyond our two to three favorite foods. Many picky eaters don't though, and their language reflects that.

Teach your child a wider food vocabulary to fill the gray area between favorites and non-preferred foods. Teach them to describe foods' tastes, textures, smells, and appearance with words that are neutral. For example, instead of "yucky" or "slimy," we could use descriptors like crunchy, dry, firm, juicy, or flavorful. Positive phrasing will help empower your child to try new foods.

Positive and neutral phrasing can also help your child prepare for new tastes. If you say, "This strawberry tastes sweet and juicy," but they don't know what those words mean, they still have no idea what to expect. If they can think about and link back to other sweet and juicy foods that they've tried in the past, they'll know how to prepare and won't feel so surprised by how it tastes or feels in their mouth.

There are many steps that you can take to empower your child and give them the tools and readiness to try new foods and continue on their adventurous eating journey!

Part Five

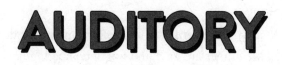

AUDITORY

Whenever I mention that our hearing is an important part of eating, people always give me funny looks. It's totally true though! For young children, their ears can be very important parts of their eating experience. Children use their auditory system to learn about foods directly. As they rip foods apart with their fingers or crunch them between their teeth, they're learning about the food's texture and how to chew it. The sound of food in their mouth can indicate how well-chewed the food is and how ready it is to swallow.

For children who are sensitive to auditory input, mealtimes can be really difficult. Mealtimes are loud and full of competing noises. Children also use their auditory sense to pick up how the adults in their lives talk about food and their eating habits. For example, if the adults in your life always call you a picky eater, you can start to believe it to be true, influencing future mealtimes. Children also learn about body image and the desirability of foods from us. We'll dive into this more in further chapters, but the way that we talk about foods directly contributes to how children feel about themselves, their food, and the people around them.

For now, consider: Does your child have difficulty following instructions or hearing you during mealtimes? Or do they seem overwhelmed, uncomfortable, or distracted by everyone's voices? This section will go over some strategies for making mealtimes more manageable for their sensitive ears so that children can be engaged and focused on trying new foods. When your child's auditory system is regulated and their sensory needs are being met, they'll be in a better place to learn about and try new foods.

16   How We Talk About Food

The way that we talk to and near our children about food will impact the way that they think about it. Even when you think they're not listening, they often are. Children hear and absorb so much, and it's important to be mindful about the ways that you talk so that your words are empowering your child.

There are some common and well-intentioned ways that I hear parents talk about food that actually contribute to picky eating rather than minimize it. I'm going to go through some of these phrases and why you might want to consider removing them from your family discussions:

Using food as a reward. "You can have this cookie after you eat your broccoli." Does that sound familiar? Sometimes it can feel like the only way to get things done. That being said, when you tell your child that they can have one food as a reward after they finish another food, it suggests that the reward food is inherently better than the other food.

After all, why would you offer a reward if the other food was just as good? We'd never say, "You can have this cookie after you eat your brownie." Just the idea of having a reward teaches your child that some foods are "better" to eat than other foods. It can also reinforce your picky eater's idea that the food on their plate isn't tasty, and they're right in preferring the dessert. This is the exact opposite of what we're trying to teach them. We want children to see the value in all foods, including healthy ones. Teach your child that all foods are worthy of exploration, and they'll be much more willing to taste them and appreciate them.

Another risk with using a desirable food as a bribe is that it can encourage children to eat when they aren't hungry so that they can get the reward at the end. This actively teaches them to ignore their body's internal cues in favor of the reward. It may also teach them to start associating food with certain emotions, like pride or frustration. Research actually shows that children that were bribed with food are more likely to be emotional eaters later on (Braden et al. 2014).

Bribery does often work in the short term. In the moment, your child may very well eat their broccoli to get to that cookie. After that though, what happens? Your child is left with the mindset that broccoli is bad and cookies are good. And the next time you offer broccoli, they're no more likely to try the broccoli than they were before.

Instead, it's helpful to present both foods equally and at the same time, letting your child make decisions from there. Presenting both (in serving sizes that you're comfortable with), sends the message that both foods are equally tasty and equally important to eat. In the long term, this makes your child more likely to want to try the broccoli at future meals. Fighting picky eating is a marathon and not a sprint, so using short-term strategies can often be counterproductive to the long-term goals.

Hiding or lying about foods. It can feel so tempting to hide cauliflower in "chicken" nuggets or carrots in macaroni and cheese. Anything to get your picky eater to eat those veggies, right? Wrong!

There's so much guilt associated with making sure that kids get the nutrients they need that sometimes hiding fruits and veggies in other foods can feel like the only way to keep children healthy. But this is another case where short-term solutions lead to long-term problems. In the short term, this strategy might help get the nutrients inside them, but in the long term, it can actually make them *pickier* rather than less picky.

Children are learning about an entirely new world of food, and they're building their ideas of food from the ground up. When children are tricked into trying new foods, it teaches them wrong information.

Instead of pretending that one food is another food, you can use the opportunity to teach your child about similarities between foods. For example, saying, "This cauliflower nugget tastes salty and savory, just like your favorite chicken nuggets!" gives them a chance to see the link between their preferred and non-preferred foods.

Teaching your child about foods truthfully is respectful. Not to say you should never combine vegetables into other foods, like black bean brownies or carrot cake, but when you do, you should involve your child in the process. This will help them learn about the deliciousness of new foods! Children are also really perceptive and frequently catch on to the fact that they're being lied to. When this happens, it reinforces the idea for them that the sneaky food is "bad." After all, why would mom or dad lie about the food if it were good?

Talking about "good" foods and "bad" foods. "This cake is so good, it's dangerous!" Does that sound familiar? Talking about foods as good or bad, dangerous, naughty, or any other judgmental word is going to shape the way that your child thinks about those foods and how they think about themselves for eating it. Do you want your child to think of themselves as naughty or bad when they have a slice of cake at a birthday party? Probably not.

At the end of the day, food is just food. Every food contains different nutrients and that's ok. It's okay to eat all foods in moderation, including those that are considered "junk" foods.

In helping your child develop a good relationship with food, it's important to teach them about the value of each food. For example, while birthday cake is full of sugar and butter, it also helps us celebrate and bond with our friends. Not to mention, it tastes good! Chips and crackers can help children develop their chewing skills, ice cream teaches children about how different temperatures feel in their mouths, and cookies can teach children how to manage multiple textures in their mouth at a time. Every food has value, and teaching your child this early can help them develop a healthy relationship with food.

When foods aren't separated into "good" and "bad," it helps prevent children from coveting certain foods and encourages them to feel comfortable with lots of foods.

"Do you like it?" This question seems innocuous right? When children try their first bite of a new or non-preferred food, our first reaction is often, "Do you like it?" This question is normally answered with an emphatic no. Why is that? In these interactions, we're speaking a totally different language than our kids are.

What we're really asking is, "What did you think about it?" but what they're hearing is, "Will you eat this every time I make it from this point forward?" So naturally their answer is going to be no! They just tried this food for the first time. Of course they don't feel ready to commit to eating it forever.

Children think that if they give us an inch, we'll end up taking a mile. They worry that if they say that they like it, they're committing to a lifetime of eating that food. And in their first couple tries, they're not ready to commit to that just yet. After all, they're still learning about it!

Instead, you could ask them something else about the experience that will get at the heart of what you hope to learn. What does that food taste like? What does it feel like in your mouth? What did you learn about this food today?

Asking open-ended questions like this will allow your child to reflect on their experience without feeling like they need to make a black and white decision about it. This will set them up for success next time!

Yes/No questions (when the answer can't be no). "Do you want some peas on your plate?" What happens if they say no? Children need to be taught that their words matter. But when we ask a yes or no question, we have to be okay with either answer.

If you put the peas on their plate anyway, it sends the message that their words and autonomy don't matter. That being said, sometimes we need to get stuff done. If you don't put the peas on their plate, then they're not getting that exposure that you've been working so hard for! So what do you do?

One strategy is to say, "*You can* put peas on your plate," instead of asking, "Do you want to put peas on your plate?"

To give them a sense of autonomy and respect while still encouraging positive behaviors, try rephrasing your questions to be more open ended. Instead of, "Do you want to take a bite?" try rephrasing to something else, like, "What do you think your next bite is going to taste like?" or, "Which food are you going to take a bite of next?" Asking questions this way provides polite encouragement and creates an opening for your child to learn and grow, without setting yourself up for failure.

You can also offer two choices that you're okay with. Instead of asking whether or not they want peas, you could say, "Do you want your peas on your plate or in your bowl?" This will give them some control in their meal, while you're still getting your mealtime goals accomplished. You could also let them help direct by asking questions, like, "Which food are you going to eat first?" This gives them control and autonomy while encouraging them toward adventurous eating.

Giving your child choices and autonomy and respecting their words will set them up for increased confidence and engagement around mealtimes and beyond.

Talking only about food. Most of these strategies are about how to talk about food during mealtimes. While that's important, talking only about food can be stressful for anxious eaters. At the end of the day, mealtimes are all about connecting, bonding, and sharing your love for one another.

While your child may need some extra dialogue around food, make sure that you continue to use this time to bond, connect, and catch up on the important things in life. Create opportunities for them to talk about their day and participate in family discussion.

In the end, the way that you talk to your child about food and mealtimes will shape their approach to food, and the thoughts and feelings they have about it, their whole life. And with some conscious effort, you can foster a sense of security and confidence through your language.

17   The Power of Crunch

Many of us grew up with our parents telling us that we needed to chew silently to have good manners. The time for good manners will come, but when your picky eater is young, loud chewing can actually be a fun and developmentally appropriate way to explore their food.

Children listen to the sounds of themselves chewing. This is one reason why children gravitate toward crunchy foods like crackers! They're an easy food to eat and they provide a lot of auditory input that tells you how well you're chewing. The sounds food makes while it's chewed (and crushed up between little fingers) give picky eaters so much information about their food. Children can't see what food looks like inside their mouth while they're eating, but they can hear it! They also know that they're done chewing and ready to swallow when the crunching noises get quieter, which is when they can avoid uncomfortable swallows.

Beyond teaching them about chewing, making crunching noises can actually motivate trying new foods. Children love to pretend to be puppy dogs or monsters devouring their food. So, as you're working with your learning eater, take turns taking bites of something—especially those crunchier foods—and pretend to chew like a dinosaur or some other animal your child likes. Loud chomping can be a particularly fun way to try new, raw vegetables or fruits.

If your child feels hesitant to take a bite of a new food, you can talk about what it might sound like in their mouth to get them excited to try. I like to ask open-ended questions or make open-ended statements, like, "I wonder what this is going to sound like when I take a bite." Building that curiosity creates space for your child to begin to wonder as well. As your child uses their auditory system to explore their food, they'll start to feel more comfortable with new foods!

18   Managing Auditory Sensitivities

For children who are sensitive to auditory input, mealtimes can be a nightmare. After all, mealtimes are often boisterous and loud, filled with talking, laughing, chewing, scraping utensils, and more. There are lots of loud and competing noises that can easily overload sensitive ears. If your child is sensitive to auditory input, read on for some strategies to keep them comfortable and engaged during mealtimes so that they'll feel confident and ready to try new foods.

When children have auditory processing differences, their difficulties can present in a number of ways:

Difficulty following instructions. Children that have difficulty with auditory processing may have trouble following instructions during mealtimes because they have trouble filtering out background noise. Do you find that your child is constantly asking you to repeat yourself? Or are you constantly asking them to set the table, and they're always ignoring you or responding, "What?" Your child may benefit from a visual reminder as well as an auditory one.

Instead of just continuing to nag and remind your child about mealtime expectations, try making a visual schedule or reminder. By writing down your expectations, your child will be able to use their visual system as well as their auditory system to process what you're asking. This makes it easier for them to follow instructions and get ready for the meal.

Responds negatively to certain noises. Does your child run screaming from the blender? Or cover their ears when the oven timer goes off? Their auditory system may be processing that as an uncomfortable noise, even if yours doesn't.

If this happens, try warning them prior to the noise so that they can prepare or go into another room. With a little bit of preparation, that noise might be less shocking and abrasive, even if they still don't enjoy it.

If that's not quite enough to mitigate the noise, you may want to consider getting your child some type of ear defenders. Ear plugs or earmuffs can help block that noise and can prevent it from being too overwhelming. Your child may alternatively like listening to music through headphones so that they can have a familiar and comforting form of auditory input to override the loud noise. To help your child become more accustomed to loud noises, you can slowly fade off their use of ear defenders over time.

Feeling overwhelmed by the noise of people talking. For children that have trouble filtering out extraneous auditory input, the sound of multiple people talking can be hard to bear. While talking at the dining table, try to ensure that only one person is talking at a time. If possible, place your child so that you're facing them and they can see your lips and make eye contact with you while you're talking. This can help keep them engaged.

If you're doing everything you can to make them comfortable and sitting with the whole family is still uncomfortable for them, set a visual time that tells them how much longer they'll be expected to sit at the table. You can slowly increase the amount of time on the timer until they're sitting with you for the whole meal.

When your child is well regulated, they'll do their best eating, learning, and communicating. If your child is uncomfortable with loud noises, competing noises, or any other form of auditory input, it can be helpful to teach them some ways to advocate for themselves and their needs. Teach them to say, "Can you please be quieter?" or, "I need to take a break because this is too loud." You can teach them to cover their ears or to leave the room if they need to. By empowering your child with extra tools, and by showing them that you're on their side, they'll know that they can handle anything mealtime throws at them.

19 Minimizing Distractions

For children with auditory sensitivities, any little noise can be a distraction. Everything from the sound of the plates scraping against the table to chairs squeaking and utensils clanking can be distracting and make it hard to focus. By minimizing these distractions, you'll make it easier for your child to handle mealtimes.

Start by taking a moment to sit at the dining table and see what small noises you can hear. Homes have all sorts of noises that most bodies tune out but that your child's body may not, like lightbulbs buzzing, dishwashers groaning, or chairs squeaking. If your child is old enough, you can ask them to tell you what they hear. Their answers may surprise you.

Once you know what sorts of noises are impacting your child, you can take steps to mitigate them. Lots of little changes could make a big difference. For example, you could place a rug under or put anti-scrape pads on the bottom of squeaky chairs.

If there are any unnecessary noises, like a clock ticking, consider removing or replacing them. Any noises that you can eliminate will make a big difference. If you often run your dishwasher during mealtimes, consider waiting until afterward. This will leave fewer noises for you to compete with while eating.

To limit distractions, you can make sure that you bring everything to the dining table before the meal starts. By the time you sit down, make sure that you have napkins, utensils, and anything else you could possibly need. Getting up and down from the table adds extra distraction and noise that your child doesn't need.

Of course, it won't be possible to entirely get rid of extra noises during mealtimes. You can take steps to try to mask outside noises. Things like white noise machines or wordless, rhythmic music can help tune out other noises.

With fewer auditory distractions, your child will be able to tune in to the things that they need to hear. They'll be more engaged with family conversation and directions and will be able to remain focused on trying new foods.

Part Six

BODY AWARENESS AND MOTOR PLANNING

(Proprioception)

Our proprioceptive system takes information from our muscles, tendons, and joints and uses that information to help us move our bodies. The proprioceptive system tells our bodies where they are in space and how we plan out motor movements. Children use their proprioception to run, jump, climb, play, and of course, to eat.

Proprioception is especially important for eating. Again, children can't see inside their mouths while they're eating. This makes it especially hard for them to plan out the motor movements associated with chewing and swallowing food. Young babies can look at their hands while they use them and learn about the sensation of movement as they watch it happen. They can't do the same with food. When they put food in their mouth, it disappears from their view, and they rely primarily on their proprioceptive system to tell them where it is in their mouth and how they're moving it.

Then, to eat, they need to coordinate over fifty muscles together to chew their food, move it backward in their mouth, and ultimately swallow it. Not to mention the muscles and motor movements required to pick up food and bring it to their mouth. And all those muscles need to work differently depending on the type of food and the size of the bite. That's a lot to coordinate!

Children use their proprioceptive systems to move food around in their mouth, chew, and swallow. If their proprioceptive system isn't functioning optimally, eating can be difficult.

Children that struggle with their proprioceptive processing may have difficulty with managing food in their mouths. This might look like putting too much food in their mouth, holding it in their cheek before swallowing, or spitting food out. Some children may take bites that are too big, or bites that are too small. It might also look like having difficulty with chewing or only accepting foods of certain textures. If they find chewing hard to coordinate, they may only eat food textures that they feel confident in managing. This can lead to picky eating. After all, why would you put something in your mouth if you didn't feel confident that you could eat it?

Luckily, there are many things that you can do to support their proprioceptive processing. First, it's important to give your child only foods that they can safely manage to eat. For young eaters, their ability to manage a food directly correlates with their gross motor skills. Children use the same muscles and core stability for both eating and *gross motor movement*—movements that use large muscles in our torso, arms, or legs—so as they become stronger, they can eat more advanced foods.

We want to make sure that we're setting up their motor planning for success by not giving them foods that are too advanced. Children that sit independently should eat smooth purees. For crawlers and cruisers, you can include solids that melt in your mouth, like crackers. For children that are walking, you can give them soft table foods, and for more advanced children that walk up and down stairs and jump, you can include hard-to-chew foods, like raw fruits and veggies.

If your child is older, talk to them about the foods that they're eating and how to chew those foods. Talking them through the process can help them gain more confidence with it. Practice biting down on something and then taking the food out of your mouth. Let them look at the teeth marks in the food. How hard do you have to bite down before you bite all the way through? Letting your child practice changing the firmness of their bite will help them think more critically about using their proprioceptive system while eating.

As your child gains more confidence with their proprioceptive system, they'll feel more confident with eating new foods as well. Improved proprioceptive processing leads to better mouth awareness and motor planning during eating.

20 Picking the Right Utensils

Picking the right utensils for your child can sound like a no brainer, but is it? There are a lot of factors to consider in finding the best utensil for your child. Armed with the right knowledge, you'll be able to set your child up for success for utensil use.

The first thing to consider is *when* you want to start offering them utensils. Most parents want their children to have polite table manners, so they start offering them as soon as possible. Despite their convenience, it's actually really important to your child's development that they start with finger feeding rather than utensils. Young children need time to use their proprioceptive system to build up their understanding of body awareness and motor planning before they use utensils.

Your child learns so much from finger feeding. They learn about their food and what the texture of that item is like. The texture on their fingers tells them what it's going to feel like in their mouth, how hard they're going to have to chew, and what they may need to do to swallow it safely. So, before you introduce your child to utensils, you want to make sure that they're confident in exploring and touching foods and have had adequate time to teach their sensory systems about their textures.

Finger feeding also teaches toddlers about the importance of where they place the food in their mouth. If they place the food on the side of their mouth, is it easier to chew than if they place it in the middle of their mouth? Think about trying to pick up and set down a pea with your fingers. You could be very precise about where you were going to set down the pea. Now what if you tried to pick it up with something long, like a pair of tongs? It would be a lot harder to be accurate! The same is true for children with utensils. They're going to be a lot more accurate in placing food in their mouth when using their fingers than when using something long, like a utensil. Practicing accurate placement teaches good mouth awareness and chewing habits, and accuracy is important because it demonstrates mastery of those skills and helps prevent choking.

You want to give your child ample time to practice self-feeding with their fingers before you introduce them to utensils. Most children are ready to use utensils around six months after they start walking. This ends up being around eighteen months old for many kids. Once children start walking, they're able to eat most foods, including those with harder-to-chew textures, like meats, and those with two or more textures, like mac and cheese and chicken nuggets.

There are many considerations in picking the right utensil, the first being what type of utensil is best to start out with. I always recommend introducing children to a spoon before a fork. Spoons are more forgiving if you overshoot or undershoot when aiming for your mouth. If you push a fork into your mouth too quickly, you could scratch yourself. With a soft-tipped spoon, you won't have that problem. Spoons are much easier to get food onto in the first place.

There are a lot of steps to eating with a spoon. You have to pick up the spoon and get a good grip on it. Then you have to find your food and put the right side of the spoon into the food, using a scooping motion to get the food onto the spoon. Then you have to pick the spoon back up, balancing it just right so that the food doesn't fall off the spoon as you aim it toward your mouth. After that you have to coordinate your awareness of where your mouth is to aim well, and open your mouth at the same time that the spoon arrives, closing it on the spoon. After you pull the spoon out, using your tongue and lips to keep the food in your mouth, you repeat it all again for the next bite.

Your child may not pick up all those steps at first. You can help your child by doing some of the steps for them. Maybe you start by getting food on the spoon and then handing it to them, or you could hold their hand to guide them through the motion of getting food onto their spoon. You know your child best and will know what type of help they'll be most receptive too. Don't be afraid to help your child in the beginning if they need it, but remember to take a step back after they've had some time to practice. After all, the goal of teaching them to use utensils is that they'll be independent with their eating, not that we have to help them with it for every bite!

Sometimes it can help to have two spoons when starting out: one for you and one for your child. This way you and your child can take turns using the spoon without fighting over it. Giving your child this independence keeps them from fighting you for control of the spoon while allowing you to move mealtime along at a reasonable pace. Plus, it helps them learn and practice before they're ready to be completely in charge of self-feeding.

You can also support your child by choosing the right spoon for them. The right spoon is going to be one that is the right size, shape, and texture.

The right spoon for a young child will be very short, around four inches long at most. I always like to think about trying to color with those giant foot-and-a-half-long pencils that many of us saw at book fairs when we were younger. It was nearly impossible to write even something as simple as our names with a big pencil like that. The extra length made precision hard, and the extra weight made our arms fatigue quickly. The same is true for toddlers with adult-length spoons. Adult-length spoons are often around the length of their entire forearm, from fingertip to elbow. Not only does this extra length add extra challenge for your child, but it's also more likely to frustrate them or cause them to choke. When introducing your child to spoons, make sure to find a very short, toddler-length spoon.

Another factor to consider in picking the right spoon is the depth of the bowl of the spoon (where the food sits). You want your child's spoon to have the shallowest bowl possible. Some spoons are even totally flat, with no bowl at all. The deeper the bowl, the harder it will be for your child to get food onto the spoon, and to get the food from the spoon into their mouth. Flatter bowls allow children to have success with dipping rather than scooping, which they may not quite have the skills for yet. Stores also sell spoons with textured bowls to help grip onto food, facilitating that learning process. While a textured bowl is a plus, it's certainly not necessary

There are so many materials that spoons are made out of, from plastic to rubber, wood to metal, and more. For the most part, the material does not matter too much, as long as it's smooth, with no hard edges. The one exception is metal. I never recommend starting a toddler out with a metal spoon for a couple reasons. First, the metal is harder and it makes it easier for children to injure themselves with it. Second, metal tends to heat up or cool down really quickly. If your child's food is warm or cool, it can change the temperature of the spoon as well, making it more likely for children to misinterpret the temperature information they're getting from the food in their mouth. Rubber, plastic, and wood spoons all tend to stay the same temperature and make it easy for children to start their journey to utensil mastery.

Once your child has mastered the spoon, they can move on to the fork. Using forks takes more precision than spoons, and your child may need help to start out. You can help by having them hold the fork in their hands and guiding their hands to poke the food and get it on the fork.

Just like using a spoon, using a fork has a ton of steps. As you're introducing your child to the fork, feel free to help them with any or all of those steps, but be sure to fade back your help quickly to support your child in being independent.

When choosing the right fork, you want to consider many of the same factors as a spoon, including size and material. You want to find a fork that is short and made out of a soft material other than metal. Children are going to need some time for trial and error—they'll make mistakes while learning about how to use a fork. You want them to have a fork that allows them to make those mistakes without hurting themselves. A fork with softer, shorter, points will allow them to practice eating without accidentally poking themselves in the face.

When introducing your child to a fork, pick soft foods that are easy to pierce with the fork's spikes. Soft foods like steamed veggies or overcooked pasta are often the best foods to start with when using forks.

Don't feel any pressure to rush your child into using utensils. Many kids don't figure out how to use utensils until between two and three years old, and that's totally fine too. The more time they have to finger feed, the more time they're spending really getting to know their food and their body.

The very last utensil to introduce your child to is a knife, and you probably don't want to do that until they're at least four or five years old. Of course, you would only allow your child to use a blunt knife at this age, but using a blunt knife can be really frustrating because it doesn't cut easily.

When you're ready to introduce your child to a knife, you can give them time to practice before introducing it at mealtimes. Let your child practice using a plastic knife on play dough, where they can practice in the context of play, so it's less frustrating. You can let your child help with food prep in the kitchen, where they can practice cutting cucumbers or tomato slices. Your child will be ready to be introduced to a knife when they can use one hand to hold the item that they're cutting and the other hand has the coordination and skill to move independently to complete the cutting motion. They'll push down with the knife to make the cut. Giving them the chance to practice with play dough or something similar will give them the confidence to try later on with food, once they're ready.

Remember that when you're introducing your child to utensils, they're likely to take much longer and be messier than they were before. That's okay! Your child is learning a new skill, and that is something to celebrate. Remember that children who observe their parents eating and using utensils tend to pick up on these skills more quickly than children who are fed away from the table. Give them the time to practice, play, and explore this new skill. With the right preparation and equipment, they'll be independently eating with utensils soon.

21 Mealtime Misbehaviors

It's important to remember that children typically misbehave for a reason. Children are learning and testing boundaries; it's a really important milestone for them to hit. That being said, it can be frustrating when children choose mealtimes (which can already be chaotic) as a time to test those limits. But by identifying the reason behind it, we can help prevent it and know how to deal with it more effectively when it does happen.

Many misbehaviors center around movement and the use of our proprioceptive system, like throwing food, getting up from the table, wiggling around in chairs, and more. Most children are frequently on the move—even more so for "sensory seekers" or children that enjoy a higher amount of proprioceptive input. When children aren't getting their sensory needs met, they can show that by trying to fulfill them themselves, by moving around in a way that feels good or by acting out in other ways to communicate their feelings of dysregulation.

With the strategies in this chapter, you'll feel more confident in staying calm through these trying moments and in preventing, managing, and correcting your child's difficult behaviors.

The first step is to think a bit about *why* your child is acting out. Children can have tricky behaviors around mealtime for all sorts of reasons. It may be that they're tired from their day and are acting out because of fatigue, or it could be that they just think it's fun to press your buttons and test those limits. Toddlers are famous for acting out because they're learning about cause and effect, or in other words, *If I do this, how will my parents react?*

But one of the most common reasons that kids misbehave is because they're anxious, dysregulated, or trying to distract from the expectations being placed on them. It feels easier to do something naughty or distracting, shifting your focus onto their behavior rather than on what food they may not be eating.

Feeling pressured to eat a new food is stressful! It can be almost impossible to take that pressure off our kids, as many of them put it on themselves, and as loving parents, we worry so much about if our children are getting enough to eat. That worry and love creates a cycle of expectation and pressure on our kids. Understanding why your child is acting out can help you approach the behavior from a place of compassion, which is key to your success. If you get angry or frustrated, the situation will escalate and get worse, but if you can stay calm and compassionate, you'll be better prepared to diffuse the situation and end their negative behaviors.

In this chapter, I'll go through some of the most common misbehaviors that I see and some ways to combat them. With all the strategies I share, remember that it can take two to four weeks to see an effect, so don't give up if it doesn't work the very first time. It's important to stay consistent once you choose a strategy to try. Any time you step back into old habits, it tells your child, "If I keep doing this long enough, my parents will eventually go back to giving me the response I want," and it can double the amount of time a strategy takes to work. If you keep it up, you'll soon see your child's negative behaviors disappearing.

Throwing food. What parent wants to clean a huge mess off the floor in addition to cooking, cleaning dishes, wiping down the kitchen, and everything else that comes with mealtime? No one! But that's part of what makes it so appealing to children.

When I picture throwing food from a child's perspective, I often think of it as dinner and a show. They're enjoying a meal, and with the minimal effort of throwing a piece of food, they get to hear the satisfying plop of food hitting the floor; they get to watch mom or dad jump up, pick up the food, and make silly, angry faces; and they get to hear all their angry commentary. Children love to feel like they can affect their parents and have control over their actions, and it's fun and inherently rewarding to have a simple activity (like throwing food) that can accomplish both.

So, while it may seem counterintuitive, the quickest way to eliminate this behavior is to refuse to play your part in the song and dance. If you ignore the throwing and refuse to get up from the table or participate in any cleanup until after mealtime, your child will get bored and stop. It can be hard at first, but the more you force yourself not to react by staying seated, keeping a neutral expression, and not saying anything, the more throwing food will lose its appeal.

On the other hand, if you've been ignoring their throwing for ages and it still continues, it's possible that it's fulfilling another need for them. The proprioceptive input from winding their arm back to throw food may feel good to their sensory system. In this case, we want to try to replace that input with another, more acceptable input.

You can try engaging them in appropriate forms of input prior to mealtimes. Maybe you can throw a ball back and forth before dinner, so they've met their throwing needs prior to mealtime. They may enjoy another form of proprioceptive-heavy play, like wheelbarrow walking or crawling through a tunnel. Through these activities, they'll be able to frontload their bodies with the input that they're craving and, hopefully, won't need to seek that input during mealtimes by throwing their food.

Excessive talking/distraction. While mealtime is meant to be a time for social gathering and bonding, some children talk too much and intend to distract from the meal. They'll talk and joke or "accidentally" drop something on the ground, all to keep the attention on something other than eating.

It can feel hard to draw the line between appropriate, social chatting and distraction chatting. My rule of thumb is that I want children to be able to finish their meal in around twenty minutes. If twenty minutes have gone by and your child still hasn't touched their plate, but they've been talking the whole time, it was probably a distraction technique.

With distraction chatting, try redirecting the conversation onto your food. You can talk about what it tastes like, the texture, the smell, or anything else about the food. Often this will shift your child's focus back onto the meal.

If your child has trouble with this and continues to redirect onto other topics, you can calmly but firmly say, "I want to talk about that with you, but let's talk about that later. Right now I'm really curious what you think about this food." This helps your child feel validated and cared for while still maintaining boundaries around appropriate mealtime conversation.

If your child is distracting by pretending to drop things, it can help to have some extras of whatever they drop readily accessible. That way you can say, "It's okay you dropped your napkin. You can leave it there, we have extras." Once your child realizes that dropping things won't delay their meal, that behavior will quickly stop.

Intentional vomiting. Gagging and vomiting can be tricky because it's such an extreme (and let's be honest, gross) reaction. Plus, it can disrupt everyone else's meal as well. There are lots of reasons why a child could be gagging or vomiting, including sensory or medical reasons, and I'd strongly encourage you to see a doctor to rule these out first. If you've ruled out any medical cause, it could be a behavior, and then these strategies would be helpful. It's not fair to use behavioral strategies for a child that doesn't have control over it though, so be sure to eliminate any other possible reasons first.

Children are smart, and many children learn that vomiting or trying to vomit can elicit a huge reaction from their parents. After all, why wouldn't it? No one wants vomit on their dining table. That being said, it becomes a problem when children are vomiting to get out of every meal.

In these instances, I like to use a "vomit bucket." This is a bucket that you keep at the dining table with you and put in front of your child when they try to vomit. The idea is that we want to minimize our reaction as much as possible. As with many other behaviors, children vomit because they learn that it will get a big reaction from their parents and will likely get them out of whatever situation they don't want to be in. In this instance, that might mean they're trying to end the meal. If we minimize our reaction as much as possible, they'll learn that their behavior isn't having its intended effect anymore, and will likely stop. Having a bucket at the dining table allows you to react as minimally as possible while still keeping the flow of mealtime going.

If your child uses their vomit bucket, try to continue with the meal as normal and end the meal when you normally would, after around twenty minutes. Vomiting can be really disruptive, but the more you are able to continue with your mealtime routine, the less your child will want to intentionally vomit.

Getting up from the table. It can be so disruptive when you sit down to a meal and your child jumps up to run into the other room. Mealtime is important family time, and it's key to have everyone sitting together for the whole meal. There are many different factors to this behavior, and different strategies to address it, depending on their age.

No matter how old your child is, there are a few things to consider. First, you want to make sure that you're always modeling good behaviors. That means *you* have to stay seated too. No jumping up to grab one more thing or running into the kitchen because you forgot something. It can help to make a "mealtime kit" with extra utensils, napkins, and serving spoons to bring to the table. That way you always have whatever you need right at your fingertips. If your child sees you getting up during mealtime, they'll feel like they can too.

Another big consideration is eliminating all distractions. What's your child going to do when they get up from the table? Do they have a favorite toy, or are they going to turn on the TV? Locking up or turning off potential distractions can help quell the urge to leave the table.

Also, make sure that their seating is appropriate for their size. Can they easily rest their elbows on the table, or is their chair too low? If they're having to work really hard to reach for food on their plate, they're going to get tired muscles and want to get up from the table sooner. With adequate support and a high-enough seat, your child will feel more comfortable at the table and want to stay there for a longer period of time.

Another consideration is whether your mealtime expectations are realistic. No child under the age of ten is going to be able to sit for an hour-long meal. While it can be relaxing for adults to eat a slow and leisurely meal, the same cannot be said for children. A fair expectation is that they need to stay at the table for twenty minutes. After this it's acceptable for them to be excused.

If your child is struggling with these expectations, their body may be looking for proprioceptive input through movement. Sitting still can be hard for children that like a lot of proprioceptive input, and they often get up and run around as a way of trying to get that input. As with other sensory-seeking behaviors, try frontloading with other, more appropriate forms of proprioceptive input. They may enjoy jumping, running, climbing, or animal walking prior to mealtimes to get their body ready to sit for fifteen minutes.

If you've set up all these routines and your child is still getting up from the table, then we can look at some age-specific strategies.

For toddlers, it may be that they would continue to benefit from being in a high chair or booster seat with a strap. They may not have the regulation skills to remain at the table just yet and may benefit from the security of feeling strapped in.

If they're in the four- to six-year-old age range, one idea is to use a visual clock or hourglass to help your child visualize how much time is left.

If your child is older than six, they clearly understand the expectations set in place for them, and you can start to use the behavior strategies that you use for other negative behaviors. It can also help to positively engage your child with a role at the dinner table. Maybe they can be in charge of serving everybody or coming up with topics for mealtime conversation. With a role and responsibility, they'll feel more engaged in the mealtime routine.

No matter their age, by making the dinner table a fun and comfortable place to be and making the rest of the house boring, your child will be more eager to stay with you.

Tantrums. Tantrums and screaming can be disruptive and stressful for everyone involved. An important thing to remember about tantrums is that they often come from a place of anxiety or dysregulation. When we feel anxious, we slip into the fight, flight, or freeze response. When we're in that mindset, we're not doing our best, upper-level thinking, with the parts of our brains that are responsible for good decision making. We're in survival mode, and those reasoning skills go out the window. That's why trying to talk children through huge tantrums doesn't work. They're just not in a place to be able to hear and understand in the same way as when they're calm. Likewise, when they're dysregulated, they're not in a place to be able to focus on what you're saying.

When your child is mid-tantrum, try to stay calm yourself. Your child will regulate off of you, and if you're anxious or stressed, your child will pick up on that and escalate. People always talk about putting your own oxygen mask on first in an emergency, and that sentiment is so true with child tantrums. Keep yourself calm, and that will keep you in a better mental place to care for your child as well. Having a plan ahead of time can help you stay regulated so that you can respond from a place of organization rather than emotion.

It's important to remember that just because your child isn't using their upper-level cognitive skills, it doesn't mean they don't hear you. Using short, simple sentences, you can remind them that they're safe and that you love them. Knowing that you're there for them will help your child calm down.

If you see a pattern to situations that trigger tantrums, I recommend finding a calm moment to discuss those with them. You can role-play with their favorite toys and problem solve with them to have some strategies that they can reach for in those harder moments. Then you can bring these strategies into your next scheduled mealtime.

The main takeaways for any challenging behavior are to stay calm, stay compassionate, and stay in the moment. It's important not to feed into their behavior and not to contribute to the cycle. Your child will model your behaviors, so if you stay calm, they'll stay calm too. No matter how frustrating they are, these tricky behaviors will pass.

22 Teaching Chewing Skills

Chewing is arguably one of the most important parts of eating. There's a big misconception that eating is something that children are born knowing how to do, that it's just an instinctive skill. Up until six months old, this is somewhat true. Children are born with a latching reflex that helps them drink breastmilk or formula when they're born. But these reflexes disappear by the time they're six months old, just in time to start eating solid foods. After this, eating skills need to be learned, and don't always come naturally. Because eating is so hard, children benefit from support from their parents in developing their eating skills.

When children learn to chew, they start with an up-and-down jaw motion as they mash the food against the roof of their mouth. As their skills advance, they'll transition to placing the food on their teeth and using an up-and-down chewing motion, also known as a vertical chew. As they transition to a more mature way of chewing, they'll use a rotary chewing movement, which includes both lateral and circular chewing movements. To try to visualize a rotary chew, consider the way a cow chews. They're experts at (the exaggerated version of) a rotary chew.

Once a child chews up their food thoroughly, they need to use their tongue to move and shape the food into a *bolus*, a ball of chewed food, in the mouth to get it ready to swallow. Once it's formed into a bolus, they'll use a wave-like motion of their tongue to move it backward in their mouth and then swallow it down.

Vertical chewing works well for soft table foods, like steamed veggies and baked fruits, but children need to master rotary chewing to be able to eat more advanced foods, like meats and uncooked fruits and veggies. When children struggle with more mature styles of chewing, they often get stuck eating only soft textured foods, or foods that melt in your mouth, like crackers

To be able to advance to more mature chewing styles, and more difficult food textures, children need two skills: they need to have the strength and coordination for the jaw movements associated with chewing, and they need to be able to move food from side to side with their tongue.

To help your child develop their coordination and strength for chewing, encourage them to practice on long, skinny teethers or foods of a similar shape. Tools that are long and skinny (picture something that's the shape of a pretzel rod), allow children to explore the back of their mouth. And it's easier to explore your mouth with something like a teether toy than it is with food, because the teether will never break up into multiple pieces like a food will when you take a bite. Teethers also have considerably less sensory involvement. They don't have any flavor or smell to distract your child from practicing their chewing skills.

With their chew toy, your child can practice large, powerful bites on it (just the way they would with food). This helps them learn to coordinate the complicated movements that they need to do with their jaw to properly chew their food.

It can be helpful to have them try holding the food still between their molars while you (or they) pull gently on the toy. Can they resist the pressure and continue to hold it? Many children like to pretend to be a dog playing tug-of-war with a bone. Holding on will build the strength that their muscles need to chew and grind up their food.

Just as important as building strength in their chewing muscles is improving the coordination of their tongue. Long, skinny teethers can be helpful for learning side-to-side tongue movement as well as building chewing muscles.

When children move a long and skinny teether or food from side to side in their mouth, it touches their tongue. Their tongue moves along the chew toy, and feeling the toy stimulates the exact movement that the mouth needs to do to move the food. Once they learn how to do that with the chew toy, they'll have the muscle memory for how to do it without. It's easier for a child to stimulate this movement with a toy, which they can control, than to make the movement with their tongue alone.

This is one benefit of babies' exploring toys with their mouth! They're practicing these skills naturally. Many children, especially those with sensory processing differences, don't orally explore toys on their own though and may prefer to avoid them. In these cases, exploring mouth toys in an age-appropriate way can build their understanding of their proprioceptive system, leading to adventurous eating and confident food exploration.

23 Ending Pocketing

Does your kiddo pocket their food? *Pocketing* is when you hold food in your mouth without swallowing it. Some families describe it as their child's "chipmunking" their food by holding it in their cheeks, sometimes for hours, before swallowing it or spitting it out. While this can feel really worrisome, it's actually very common, and there are several things we can do to fix it.

First, it's important to think about why children pocket their food. This can come down to several different reasons.

For many children, their proprioceptive system isn't effectively processing the sensation of having food in their mouth. For children that like high amounts of proprioceptive input, they may enjoy that feeling of pressure on the inside of their cheeks from the food. That pressure may feel soothing, and they may hold that food in their mouth to continue that sensation.

On the other hand, their sensory systems may not be registering the pressure correctly, and they may not even realize that it's there! If your body has difficulty registering input and pressure, it may not notice mashed, warm food. For undiscerning sensory systems, pocketed food can feel very similar to saliva, and because of this, they may ignore it.

A third reason is that some children hold food in their mouth when they don't like it. This can feel sort of counterintuitive, right? After all, if you don't enjoy a food, why would you hold onto it rather than swallowing it down? We do the exact same thing as adults though. Have you ever taken a bite of your great aunt's horrible, dry meatloaf and found yourself chewing and chewing and chewing? It can be hard to bring yourself to swallow something that your sensory systems find uncomfortable, and the same is true for kids!

Conversely, this can also happen when they do enjoy the texture, but don't have the oral motor skills to chew it adequately. If the texture is too difficult, they may continue working on it until their mouth gets tired, when they take a break from chewing and pocket instead.

Are their chewing skills driving pocketing? Take a look at their pocketed food once they spit it out. How chewed up is it? If it looks thoroughly chewed up, then they probably had the skills to chew it and instead are having difficulties with the sensory-processing aspect of eating.

Most children pocket because of the way that their proprioceptive system registers the food. Either they enjoy that sensation of extra pressure or they aren't registering the feeling at all. The solution to both is the same. We want to frontload their eating experience with some extra sensory input to their mouth. The extra input will help fulfill that need for the extra mouth pressure so that they don't need to rely on pocketing to get that sensation. It will also increase their awareness and arousal around their mouth, so that they're better able to notice foods inside their mouth and don't forget about them and turn to pocketing.

To encourage them to pocket less often, we want to help give more sensory input to the inside of their mouth while they're eating. We can do that through a number of ways. The easiest ways to provide them this input are through harder textures, vibration, cold temperatures, and stronger flavors.

If your child has the chewing skills for them, you can start by including crunchy foods in each meal. Crunchy foods are harder in texture, and chewing them takes more mouth muscles than softer foods. They create more pressure between your teeth with each bite, and that pressure translates to increased sensory input. By alternating between the crunchy and soft foods on their plate, your child will be able to better regulate their awareness of their mouth and will more pocket less often.

Vibration is another strong form of input. I like to use vibrating toothbrushes because these tend to be more readily available, but there are vibrating oral motor tools available as well. Using a vibrating toothbrush before meals will help your child frontload the input that they need to ready their mouth for eating. The vibration from the toothbrush wakes up those muscles and helps facilitate more efficient swallowing to prevent pocketing.

Foods with colder temperatures can discourage pocketing. Offering a side of frozen fruit or veggies can wake up your child's mouth muscles between bites of warmer foods. The colder temperatures activate muscles and remind those chewing muscles to keep working. The colder temperatures also help your child's sensory systems differentiate the food in their mouth from their saliva, further encouraging them to swallow efficiently.

To increase their mouth arousal, you can flavor their food more strongly, if they enjoy those flavors. Flavoring our food with spices or sauces helps us know where food is in our mouth more clearly, which encourages efficient swallowing as well.

You can also help your child stop pocketing by coaching them through it. Remind them to take small bites rather than overload their mouth with too much food. The smaller volumes will be easier to manage and efficiently swallow.

Additionally, you can encourage them to drink as needed. Carbonated beverages can be extra beneficial for this, as the bubbles can wake up their mouth's sensory systems as well. Using an open cup for drinking is most practical because the way that the mouth closes around the lip of the cup results in their drink flooding into their mouth. This helps clear the food from all corners of the mouth, as opposed to straw or sippy-cup drinking, which may make it easier to hold onto pocketed food.

There are many strategies that can help your child decrease their pocketing, but not every strategy will work for every child. It can take some trial and error to figure out what strategies your child and their sensory system respond to best. In the meantime, try to stay calm and remain consistent with your child. Though it can be stressful, you want to avoid getting too frustrated with your child so that it doesn't turn into a game or a fun way for them to get attention. Armed with the strategies from this chapter, your child's pocketing days will soon be over.

Part Seven

BALANCE
(Vestibular System)

Our vestibular system is our balance system. It tells us how our body is attached to our head: is it leaning forward, backward, or sideways? It helps us coordinate balance and movement together and works closely with our proprioceptive (body awareness) system for this.

We get the information for our vestibular system from our inner ear. In our inner ears, we have tubes, called semicircular canals, and in those tubes are fluid and little pieces of calcium carbonate, called otoconia. The fluid flows to an area of our inner ear called our ampulla, which has little hairs that move in response to the fluid. There are three sets of semicircular canals that tell us about when our head is nodding up and down, tilting side to side, or shaking left and right as though you were shaking your head no. As the tubes tilt, the fluid moves and with it moves the otoconia. The otoconia stimulate little hairs in the tubes, telling your body about how it's moving. They also stimulate the little hairs in the ampulla. These little hairs gather information about the direction and the speed that the fluid is moving in and tell the brain what's going on with your balance.

I like to think of the canals and crystals in our ears like half-full water bottles with several little rocks inside it. As you move and shake the water bottle, the water sloshes back and forth and moves against the inside of the water bottle, moving the little rocks (or otoconia) with it. When the tube has an appropriate amount of liquid, the fluid and rocks both flow smoothly, and you can hear the sloshing noise of the fluid inside the water bottle.

We can run into problems if there are issues that prevent the fluid from moving smoothly—as with ear infections, for example. When this happens, the water doesn't flow as efficiently and doesn't move the little rocks in the same way. This can cause the dizzy feeling that you experience with ear infections. If your child gets chronic or frequent ear infections, this may be impacting their balance and comfort level with their mealtime seating.

Regardless of how effectively your child is processing their vestibular sense, the input that they get from it can be hugely important during eating. Children's sense of balance affects their security while sitting at the table. It affects their core stability, which in turn affects their chewing skills, attention, and willingness to sit at the table. Read on for more ways to use your child's vestibular system to set them up for success at the dinner table.

24 Positioning and Posture

Many people assume that high chairs and dining chairs put your child in an optimal position for eating, but that's unfortunately not always true. As a feeding therapist, I would say that the majority of the seating setups that I see are actually not ideal. It can be hard to find a good chair that adequately supports and positions your child.

Inadequate positioning negatively affects children's balance and vestibular processing. If your child isn't adequately supported, their balance will be thrown off, and they'll wiggle. Poor support decreases their endurance for sitting and increases their distraction levels, making it harder for them to stay still while eating. Unsteady seating can also leave them at higher risk for choking. When your child has a harder time sitting still for mealtimes, they'll have a harder time focusing and learning to eat. So what do you look for in good mealtime seating?

Foot support. It's important that your child have adequate support for their feet. We want their knees to be at a ninety-degree angle, with their feet flat and pressed firmly against the foot rest. Think about when you, as an adult, sit at a high bar stool or another chair where your feet can't touch the ground. What's the first thing that your feet do when you sit down? They slide back until they find a part of the chair that they can rest on. As adults, we never let our feet swing while we're eating, and we should make it the same for our children. They need that foot support to give their bodies the stability to eat safely. Wiggling while eating increases the risk of choking, and adequate food support gives bodies the stability to eat safely. When looking at how to pick a mealtime chair, you want to make sure that, if their feet can't reach the ground, you provide a footrest. If you are concerned that your child may stand up on their foot rest, putting them at risk for falling, you can use a seat belt, tray, or close supervision to ensure their safety.

With how quickly children grow, it can be helpful to find a chair with an adjustable footrest. If you can't, or those high chairs are unaffordable, you can make a footrest out of a cardboard box or shoebox. Place the box where their feet go and anchor it for stability. If your child's chair has a foot rest but it's too low for their feet to reach, you could raise it a couple inches by cutting a piece of a pool noodle to attach to the top. If you're feeling crafty, you can even make a footrest out of wood or any other solid material. Having a footrest will greatly improve your child's trunk stability while they're eating.

Trunk support. Another thing to look at in your child's positioning in their chair is what their torso is doing. Are they slouching or leaning back? Or do they have an upright posture? For ideal positioning, we want our children to have their hips at a ninety-degree angle and sit straight up, with their back fully supported. The back of your child's chair will extend to the top of their back, or even the top of their head, and will allow them to rest their full back on the back of the chair while keeping their hips at ninety degrees. If your child is too small for their chair, you can put a folded beach towel behind or next to your child until they're supported at all sides and in a good position. Adding the towel helps fill in the gaps between your child and the chair and gives them the support that they need to focus on safe eating.

Adequate support and posture during eating is really important, especially for new eaters. Learning to eat is really difficult. Your child is learning to use new muscles and to coordinate complex movements of their mouth muscles. They're also likely challenging themselves to interact with or try a new food. If they're wobbly while sitting, or are having to focus on keeping their stomach muscles engaged, they won't have their full focus on eating. Learning to eat can be hard, so we want to give them the stability and support they need to give eating their full attention. Without adequate torso support, eating takes way more energy than it needs to. As a result, children that eat unsupported may tire quickly and end their meal prematurely. Some may even skip meals entirely if they're feeling too challenged by the seating.

If your child's chair doesn't provide enough torso support, it increases the odds that your child will wiggle and have a hard time sitting still. Your child may scoot back and forth inside their high chair, making them distracted and making eating hard to focus on. I often hear parents tell their children, "Sit up straight," or, "Don't lean on the table." Before you give them cues like that though, make sure that they have the trunk support to be able to follow through on what you're asking. Without a chair that provides adequate support, your child may not be able to maintain a good position and may have to lean on the table or slouch during their meal to support themselves.

Table or tray height. The last thing that you want to look at is the height of the table or your child's tray (if they're using a high chair). The goal is that their eating surface will hit just above their belly button, so that their elbows can rest on the table while at a ninety-degree angle. This position ensures that they can comfortably reach their food without having to lift their arms up significantly. It also allows them to have a good view of all the food on their tray, so they can interact with, learn about, and eat all the food available to them, increasing the success of any food introductions or experiences.

Mealtimes often induce stress in picky eaters, as they're being asked to try something new or daunting. They may be looking for any possible distraction or reason to leave the table. If their chair does not adequately support their positioning, the way that their body wiggles may provide an easy and fun distraction from the mealtime, taking away from your ultimate goal of encouraging them to try a new food. With adequate positioning, they'll have an increased tolerance for sitting at the table and will be more likely to eat well and try new foods.

In summary, your child's ideal mealtime position is with their elbows, hips, knees, and ankles all at ninety degrees. If this is hard to picture, imagine the corner of a square. You want your children to have their backs supported, sitting up straight, their knees even with their hips, and their feet supported and firmly under them. In this positioning, they'll be ideally situated to have a positive mealtime experience.

25 Setting Mealtimes Up for Success

Our vestibular system tells us about how our body is moving and shifting. It affects our posture, movement, balance, coordination, attention, and sensory arousal. Children's vestibular processing helps them remain focused, engaged, and seated at the table during mealtimes. It also helps them stay in a secure position with an open airway for safe eating. If your child's vestibular processing isn't supporting their eating, there are steps you can take to set them up for success.

Some children are extra-sensitive to vestibular input. These children often avoid activities where they need to shift their center of balance. Small movements can feel overwhelming to their bodies. For these children, climbing into a high chair or dining chair can feel daunting. After all, if your balance is off, the last thing you're going to want to do is to climb away from the floor. It can feel scary, like you might fall! For these children, positioning is key. Helping them feel secure during mealtimes will allow them to feel safe while eating. If your child reports feeling unsafe in their seating arrangement, even with a footstool, they may feel more secure in a height-appropriate chair. This way they can plant their feet firmly on the floor rather than on a footstool. For children that are extra-sensitive to vestibular input, they may feel more confident closer to the ground. If your child is sensitive to vestibular input, developing a secure mealtime position for them will be key to increasing their comfort during mealtimes.

Some children are undersensitive to vestibular input. This means that their body either isn't adequately recognizing vestibular input or prefers higher amounts of vestibular input but needs more input to help them regulate. Undersensitivity can present in different ways. Some children have bodies that register only a fraction of the input that they get. They have a dampened sensory system and can appear very passive or have a hard time interacting with their environment. This might look like having difficulty staying upright in their chair, leaning on the table, or sliding onto the floor.

Children that are undersensitive to vestibular input can alternatively become sensory seeking, where their bodies recognize that they aren't getting enough input and respond by trying to seek that out. These children are often described as "always on the go." They may have a hard time sitting still for meals, because they're constantly moving around to try to regulate their vestibular systems. Sometimes these children prefer to graze, snacking throughout the day, rather than sit for fifteen to twenty minutes for a meal, because remaining sedentary for that long is uncomfortable for them.

If your child falls into one of these undersensitive categories, you can support them by finding more efficient ways to get the input that they need to feel regulated before—rather than during—the meal. When your child is running around the house, they're getting small amounts of vestibular input. This can mean that it takes a long time for them to build up to the amount of input that their body wants to feel regulated. If you help them to participate in more vestibular-heavy activities, children may be able to regulate more rapidly so that they're able to sit and focus during mealtimes. If they're set up for success prior to the mealtime, they're more likely to be willing to try new foods.

When you're planning vestibular activities for your child, remember the three planes of movement: side to side, up and down, and twisting like you're shaking your head no. For example, swinging on the swing involves up-and-down movement, and swaying to music might include side-to-side movement. Spinning while on a swivel chair would include twisting movement.

Track your child's response to movement in each plane. Some children find movement in one plane to be relaxing, while others can be too exciting. With some tracking and intentional play (or expert advice from your child's occupational therapist), you can plan regulating activities for prior to mealtimes.

Before mealtimes, try involving your child in play that includes a lot of movement and balance shifting. Many children like jumping on the trampoline, crawling through a tunnel, swinging either on a swing or in a blanket held by adults, walking like animals, or playing Ring Around the Rosie. Of course, every child has different preferred activities—you'll want to personalize the activities that you choose for their individual interests.

Including these activities prior to mealtimes will give your child the input that they're seeking when they run around the house or wiggle in their chair during mealtimes. With their vestibular needs met, they'll be better able to sit still and focus on eating and trying new foods.

Part Eight

INTERNAL BODY CUES (Interoception)

Interoception is our body's interpretation of internal body cues, like hunger, fullness, thirst, needing to go to the bathroom, and many more. I think of it as the invisible wizard that does a lot of the magic of eating behind the curtains. Though it's not as obvious a sense as some of our others, it's integral in the process of eating. Because our interoception tells us when we're hungry, thirsty, and full, it's the sense that motivates eating and trying new foods. If your child's body isn't accurately reading these cues, of course they're going to be less motivated to eat. There are many things that can impact your child's understanding of their hunger and fullness cues, including reflux, constipation, or other medical concerns that can make eating less comfortable. If your child is having discomfort with eating or is straining to defecate, they may be less likely to want to eat.

From a mealtime routine and family dynamic perspective, there are things that we do as parents that negatively impact children's understanding of their interoceptive processing. Habits like encouraging them to clear their plate or eat when they aren't hungry can send the message that they should ignore their body's cues. Over time this can dampen or confuse the signals that their body is getting!

Luckily, though, we can help make sure that they're getting clear cues from their body so that they're best able to interpret their interoceptive sense.

26 Teaching Your Child to Read Their Body Cues: Hungry or Full?

Teaching your child to understand what their body is saying is one of the best things that you can do for them. Understanding body cues seems like something that we should all just innately understand from birth, but things like stress, feeling rushed, and body image can get in the way. Factors like these can make listening to our body hard for us as adults and for our children too. Children are still learning about their bodies, and they require even more support to develop healthy relationships with them. A better understanding of hunger and fullness can support overall wellness, positive body image, and better eating. But how do you support your child in developing a good understanding of hunger and fullness feelings?

First, it's important to understand how our body interprets those cues. It can take about twenty minutes for food to reach our stomach and for our body to register feeling satisfied. So if we're rushing through a meal, it can be easy to overeat. When we eat quickly, we often continue eating past when our stomach would tell us that it's totally full. This confuses our brain and makes it harder for our brain to understand what fullness feels like.

Children often can't sit for a long period of time. We expect mealtime to take no longer than twenty to thirty minutes for children, regardless of their age. Any longer than that and they can fatigue, which will negatively impact their eating and their willingness to try new foods. It can also impact the way that their bodies process and understand those feelings of hunger and fullness. After the start of a mealtime, it typically takes twenty minutes for the brain to start sending out fullness cues. If your child is sitting at the table for longer than twenty to thirty minutes, they likely aren't eating very much by then because their stomach is full. If they *are* still eating, sitting longer at the table and continuing to eat after the feelings of fullness have set in could negatively impact their understanding of those cues.

Your child's stomach is about the size of their fist. That's tiny, right? Children don't have much room in their stomachs, so they tend to get full quickly. Their portion sizes can look miniature compared to ours as adults, and it can feel like they're not getting enough to eat. You should trust your child to eat what they need to. Their stomach is small, so their serving sizes will be too. If your child is having difficulty gaining weight and isn't able to regulate this on their own, consider talking with your medical team to further navigate this.

Most children, though, may start to feel full after what seems like a very small serving size, and this can be enough to support their body and growth. It can be hard to decide what the right serving size is for your child. Instead of trying to decide yourself, let your child decide what's right for their body. Encourage them to take a small first serving and to get additional servings if they want them. This way they'll pause between servings and listen to their body, deciding if they really want more or if they're full. If a large serving goes on their plate to start out, they may feel pressured to finish the whole portion, which can lead to over- or undereating.

Regardless of how much your child eats, as a parent, you should refrain from commenting on it. Praising your child for clearing their plate, or berating them for the opposite, puts pressure on your child to base their food intake on what's put on their plate rather than what their body is telling them. Having rules about clearing plates has actually been shown to contribute to obesity later in life (Robinson, Aveyard, and Jebb 2015). Letting your child determine how much they want to eat helps them develop a healthy relationship with both food and their body, and this goes for children as well as for adults. Commenting on how much someone ate, regardless of the amount, can make them feel self-conscious and can create anxiety. Let your child be in charge of interpreting and communicating with their own stomach.

Because children's stomachs are small and their energy levels are huge, they need to eat frequently to get their nutritional needs met. It's typical for a child on solid foods to eat three meals and two to three snacks a day. You want your child to have at least two hours between when you offer food so that their stomach has time to clear and they can experience that hunger sensation. Giving them two hours between meals and snacks will allow their stomach to make room for new food, but not make them so hungry that they're uncomfortable. When your child is hungry, they're more likely to try new foods, eat more, and have a successful meal.

The topic of snacks brings me to one of the biggest distractors from a good appetite for toddlers and young children: milk. While milk is important for meeting our calcium needs—especially in youngsters—many children continue to drink too much milk as they get older, which can significantly impact the appetites of older toddlers. According to the American Academy of Pediatrics, most children two years of age and up should be drinking only around two cups of milk a day (2011). If your child is drinking significantly more than that by that age, they're going to fill up on milk and have no room left in their stomach for any solid food. If this sounds like your child, consider talking to your medical team about the appropriate amount of milk for your child's specific weight, height, and nutritional needs, and how to manage their nutrition while weaning down to the recommended daily volume of milk.

If your child is drinking only the recommended amount of milk but you still feel like it might be negatively impacting their appetite, consider when you're giving it to them. Milk is full of protein, which can be a good thing, but it means that it's really filling. If you're giving your child milk within two hours before a meal, they're likely full on milk. Remember, their stomach is only the size of their fist. If there's a cup of milk in there, it doesn't leave much room for their solid foods. Consider giving your child their milk with their meal, or even after it, instead of before. This will allow them to fill up on solid foods and will ensure that they have an appetite for trying new foods during the mealtime, rather than start the meal with a belly full of milk.

You can support your child in understanding their hunger and fullness feelings by encouraging mindful interaction and conversation during meals. Make sure to unplug from all technology and remove distractions. If your child is focused on a screen or toy, they're not thinking mindfully about their food or their body. Be sure to model mindful eating for them as well. Talk to them about what hunger and fullness feel like. Encourage them to think about the different feelings they get when they're hungry versus full. How does their head feel? Clear or cloudy? How does their body feel? Strong or shaky? How does their stomach feel? Empty or firm? Our bodies give us lots of different cues to indicate what our food needs are, and as soon as your child is old enough to talk, you can start talking to them about what those signals feel like.

It's important to note that feeling hungry is different than feeling a craving for something. We feel hungry when our stomachs are empty and we need food. We can feel cravings for a bunch of reasons. It could be because we smelled something, saw an advertisement for something, remembered a favorite meal, or even saw someone eating something else. Cravings are our body's way of saying, "I want to taste that," and our body can have that thought whether or not we're hungry. Teach your child the difference between cravings and hunger. While it's not bad to give in to cravings, we want to teach our children to listen to their bodies about how much food they should be putting in.

On that note, children's appetites can vary quite a bit, from day to day or even hour to hour. As a parent, it's easy to feel the pressure and expectation that your child is going to eat the same quantity at every meal. That's not how it works though! Children's nutritional needs vary drastically and frequently, based on their activity level, how they're growing, and their overall development. Some days they'll be really hungry and others they won't, and both are okay. It can be scary to think about, but it's 100 percent okay and normal for your child to only pick at some meals. Most children will have one great meal per day and pick at the rest of their meals. If your child eats lightly, or even skips a meal, they'll make up those calories sometime in the next twenty-four hours. You can help your child honor their body cues by accepting when they want to eat less or more.

Another way to guide our children toward developing good awareness of their hunger and fullness sensations is to keep mealtime to the table. When children graze—intersperse mealtime with playtime and wander around the house—it can take hours to eat one meal. When your child is grazing, they're constantly putting just enough food in their stomach not to be overly hungry, but they're never allowing themselves to feel full either. Instead, try limiting solid foods two hours before a meal and limiting liquids one hour before a meal (as long as it doesn't make your child dehydrated). This allows their stomach to have time to clear so that they're ready to eat by the time their meal is ready. We want to set our children up for success during mealtimes so they approach food with a desire and willingness to eat.

If your child is grazing all day long on food, juice, or milk, they're not letting their body ever experience hunger. Hunger can feel like this big, scary concept, but it's a totally normal feeling that your child needs to learn about. If we overprotect our children from feeling hunger, their bodies will never signal that they need food. Without experiencing hunger, your child will never be able to learn how to identify those cues for themselves. Your child needs to learn how to communicate with their body to have a healthy relationship with it.

You can help your child understand hunger and fullness by teaching them to see food for what it is (sustenance) rather than what it's not (a coping strategy, emotional regulation, etc.). To teach this, try not to use food as a bribe. Saying things like, "If you're good at the store, I'll give you a cookie," creates the idea that food is a goal, a reward, or a prize. It puts food on a pedestal and gives it connotations that can confuse your child's awareness of their body.

A healthy relationship with food is important to model in your own life as well. If you use food to cope with a hard day at work or a stressful interaction with a family member, your child will too. If you berate yourself for taking that second slice of pie, your child will too. Set a healthy example for your child, one that you want them to follow. Food isn't supposed to be something that's tied to our self-worth. It's how we take care of our bodies and how we enjoy our culture. Food doesn't have to be just for sustenance.

It can be for joy, memories, family, and friends. We want our children to listen to their bodies and have a healthy relationship with food rather than depend on it as a coping strategy. Helping your child develop a good relationship with food is a gift that will last a lifetime.

To support your child in understanding their body cues, set a good routine and listen to your child and their body cues. Try to take pressure and expectations off your child and yourself. They've got this! And if they make mistakes, that's okay. They're still learning about their bodies, and part of learning is making mistakes. With a good routine and some good modeling, your child will learn to respect and take care of their body in a healthy way.

27 Managing Constipation

One common issue that can affect children's willingness to eat and try new foods is constipation. When a child is constipated, their body sends them a signal that says, "We're all full down here—don't send any more food!" This can strongly affect their appetite. Constipation is incredibly common, affecting about 20 percent of people (Harris et al. 2006).

Children should defecate at least once daily so that they're getting accurate hunger and fullness cues. Constipation can mess with a child's ability to understand when they're hungry or full, and this leads to food refusal or decreased appetite.

A number of things can cause constipation, like changes in routine or diet, anxiety, or not enough liquid intake. Constipation can also be a side effect of medications. If your child struggles with constipation, consider tracking their symptoms and diet to see if there's a correlation. Maybe they always get constipated after the weekends, when your family is more likely to go out to eat, or maybe they notice it's difficult to defecate a day or two after eating cheese-heavy meals, like pizza. Finding these patterns can be key for addressing the root cause of their constipation. Your child's medical team can be a great resource for this, so if you're feeling stuck, don't be afraid to ask for help!

If your child isn't defecating at least once per day, or they're straining, or the texture of their stool is hard, then your child's constipation is likely impacting their appetite. There are lots of things you can do to help your child with constipation.

One of the easiest habits to modify in your routine is to encourage your child to drink more water. Having water readily accessible throughout the day and at mealtimes can make defecating easier. If your child doesn't like water, try including a small amount of juice in it for flavoring. I like to use prune or pear juice because these juices naturally help with constipation. Children can also be motivated to drink through fruit ice cubes. Freezing fruit can make their water feel fancy and can add some flavoring as well.

Modifying their cup can help increase fluid intake. Consider letting them pick a motivating, themed cup or straw. Silly straws and cups can make drinking novel and fun and can encourage better drinking habits. If these aren't motivating for your child, another idea is to put a rubber band on their cup as a fun challenge. Who can drink to the rubber band line first? Teaching your child to enjoy water will set them up with healthy habits for life while helping their constipation.

Increasing your child's fiber intake can also ease constipation. If you feel that fiber intake may be to blame for your child's constipation, consider reaching out to your doctor about this. As your child learns to become a more adventurous eater, they may naturally eat more fiber in their daily routine. Different types of fiber can have different effects on constipation though, and if used incorrectly, can make it worse instead of better. Any rapid changes to fiber intake can cause gastrointestinal discomfort, gassiness, and bloating, so it's important to make slow changes under the supervision of your medical team.

When looking at your child's diet, consider adding in certain foods that naturally relieve constipation. Prunes and pears contain a natural laxative, sorbitol, which can help with hard stool. Eating a small amount of prunes and pears each day can alleviate their symptoms.

Take a look at your child's dairy consumption as well. Dairy can be constipating. Many children, especially picky eaters, are drawn to milk as a favorite beverage and drink large quantities of it a day. If your child drinks more than the recommended volume for their age per day, you may want to consider limiting it or switching to water.

Last, but certainly not least, keeping your child active can alleviate constipation. Having one hour of active play time each day can help keep things moving through their digestive system. The contraction of muscles and increased blood flow during exercise will help with constipation as well.

With any of these remedies, remember that they have longitudinal effects. You likely won't see any changes on the very first day of incorporating a new change. These changes can take days or weeks to build up and have a cumulative effect over a number of days. Your medical team can be a good resource when deciding what changes you may need to incorporate into your child's routine, but addressing any potential constipation will make sure that your child's digestive system is sending clear cues to their interoceptive system.

28 Raising a Child That Eats Intuitively

Being in tune with your interoceptive system means that you eat when you're hungry and stop when you're full, listening to your physical cues about food. This awareness leads to a healthier, more natural, and balanced relationship with food.

The wonderful thing about interoceptive eating for children is that most children are born instinctually knowing how to regulate their food intake! When babies are born, they cry when they're hungry and stop eating when they're full. They're in tune with their body's needs, and as they eat, they're wholly focused on their meal.

As we get older though, it gets harder to listen solely to our bodies about what and how much to eat. There's pressure from media and often from friends and family to lose weight. During mealtimes there are distractions—like watching television, organizing homework, chasing the dog away from the table, and so many more—that limit our ability to focus on our internal cues. To help raise your child to maintain the ability to listen to their body, you can foster and model healthy habits related to food, both physically and psychologically.

Because being in tune with your body means consistently checking in with your interoceptive system during meals, it's helpful to always start with small portions of meals and allow your child to get additional helpings during mealtimes. This means never making your child clear their plate but rather letting them be in charge of how much they want to eat. Being in charge of portion size teaches your child to honor their own hunger and fullness cues and to listen to them during mealtimes.

If your child is trying to decide if they want to get more food, you could help them talk through the thought process of listening to their interoceptive cues. Try asking them, "How does your stomach feel?" or, "What is your stomach saying?" Questions like these will help form their internal monologue around mealtimes and their interoception.

On top of how much to eat, interoception also signals what nutrients you're craving. Honoring interoceptive cues for what to eat will help your child find satisfaction in their food. However, because they're children, they don't always have the ability to translate a craving into a concrete need. For example, if their body is craving calcium, their limited experience and exposure might steer them toward processed crackers instead of healthier or more nutritionally complete alternatives. They're not ready to plan a healthy meal, and they need their parents' expertise to help them find foods that contribute to a healthy diet. You get to decide what to serve for dinner, but they get to decide how much they put in their mouths. As they mature, they'll learn to associate the satisfaction they get from food with the healthy foods they chose to eat off their plate (Satter 1990).

You can teach your child to find satisfaction in exercise. Teach your child to exercise because they like the way their body feels rather than because they need to burn calories. Show them the fun in kicking a ball around or climbing on the playground. It can be even better to find activities that the family can do together, like having dance parties, going for walks, or playing catch.

You can also model healthy language surrounding food and their body. Diets tend to label foods as "good" or "bad," when in reality foods are just foods. Each one contains some amount of protein, carbohydrate, or fat, and we need all of these to survive. Assigning worth to them likewise assigns worth to the people that eat those foods. You aren't a bad person for eating "bad" foods, and the last thing we want to do is associate shame or negativity with certain foods. Each food has value and is "good" in some sense. Of course, we don't want to eat donuts for every meal, but all foods in moderation are okay. It's better to teach your child to find the joy in eating vegetables in their own right than to say we have to eat them because they're healthy. Teach your child the joy of grilling an ear of corn outside, or the fun of sampling different spices on their zucchini, rather than turn vegetable eating into a chore.

This language extends to your body as well. Try not to talk negatively about your body, or draw attention to the appearance of specific body parts. Rather than talk about the size or appearance of your body, you can instead talk about how you like your body for what it lets you do. It lets you carry your child, soak up the sun at the beach, and play board games with your family. Or, don't talk about your body at all! We're so much more than the shape of our bodies, and wouldn't you rather your child learn to love themselves for their heart and compassion than the way their body looks?

It's important that you try to model these behaviors, though it can be easier said than done, as several decades of diet culture have shaped many people's thoughts about food. However, if you're dieting, talking about your body in negative ways, or restricting what you eat, your child is going to pick up on that and internalize those beliefs themselves. It can be worth reflecting on your own thoughts about food and your body. Are these beliefs serving you and benefitting your life? If they aren't, ask yourself what you want to pass on to your child. Protecting and fostering their sense of interoceptive eating will last them a lifetime.

Part Nine

MENTAL HEALTH

The ways that we perceive food, eating, and their effects on our bodies are strongly linked to our skills in eating and trying new foods. Children learn how to think and feel about food and their bodies from their parents, so it's important to support your child's psychological, as well as their sensory, approaches to eating. In fact, it's been found that the interplay between anxiety and sensory sensitivities can impact children's picky eating (Zickgraf and Elkins 2018).

Trying unfamiliar or non-preferred foods can be scary and daunting, and many picky eaters face this challenge frequently. Empowering your picky eater is important so that they feel ready to confidently approach new foods. The coming chapters will teach you how to support your child through anxious moments and how to model positive psychological self-care for them.

Picky eating can draw a lot of attention to the foods that your child eats, and may, even unintentionally, put more emphasis on their body shape or size. Unfortunately, body image concerns are quite prevalent in children, even as young as preschool. Regardless of your child's weight, they deserve to love, cherish, and celebrate their body. The following chapters will help you guide your family through positive lifestyle changes while teaching your child to love themselves and the body that they're in. In supporting your child's mental health, you'll steer them toward happy, healthy, successful, and adventurous mealtimes.

29 Food and Anxiety

Anxiety is something that many picky eaters have, especially around food. Children might have anxiety about trying new experiences, about what something will taste or feel like, or just about the expectations on mealtimes in general. Parenting a picky eater is stressful. You worry about if your child is getting the nutrients they need to learn, grow, and flourish. You worry about their getting picked on by other kids for their preferences. You worry about their going hungry while at school. The worry list is endless, and children notice those worries and often place that negativity on themselves, even if we don't mean for it to happen. So how can we break the cycle of anxiety and nervousness and make eating fun?

First, it's important to think about the difference between adaptive (healthy) anxiety and disordered (unhealthy) anxiety. Everyone, children and adults alike, experiences anxiety to some extent, and this doesn't have to be a bad thing. *Adaptive anxiety* is something we evolved to have to keep us safe. It tells us when a situation is unsafe and gives us the rush to get ourselves back to safety. For example, we feel nervous when we almost end up in a car accident. Our bodies immediately respond, increasing our heart rate and speeding up our body's reactions, to enable us to turn quickly and get out of the way of an oncoming car. The problem is when our bodies have responses that are disproportionate to the situation that they're in, or don't resolve once we're safe. When our bodies continue to feel unsafe after the threat is over or when they deem a safe situation unsafe, we begin to have *disordered anxiety*. Many of our picky eaters feel genuine fear and anxiety when it comes to trying new or non-preferred foods. It can be easy to say, "Why don't you just try it?" or, "I know if you tried it you would end up liking it," but from our children's perspectives, it's not that easy. These foods represent a real and genuine fear in their minds, and sometimes it reaches the point where even sitting at the table can feel threatening because they know they're going to be exposed to something they aren't comfortable with. The key is understanding their anxiety and setting up the situation so that your child understands their feelings and moves past them.

Something to understand as a parent is that anxiety and calm are both contagious. If you are feeling stressed about your child and their eating, they're going to pick up on that and feel anxious too. We need to make sure to meet our children where they are and to exude the feelings that we want our child to feel. Food and family routines around food are supposed to be fun, culturally rich, family oriented, and relaxing. We need to make sure that we're leading our child toward experiencing that goal by being a good model. Calm breeds calm. When you're supporting your child through feeding, it's important to remember to be consistent. When your child knows what to expect from your routine, that eliminates the unknown. A consistent routine will help your child feel more at ease and more in control of their feeding experience. When routines are predictable, they feel safer and our anxiety decreases. With calm and consistency, your child will be ready for you to help guide them through their anxiety toward feeling more adventurous with food.

It can be easy to let your child's preferences and restrictions change or limit your family's meals and mealtime routines. With picky eaters, it's often easier not to pick the fight and to just give them something that you know they'll eat. No one wants each mealtime to be a battle, but accommodating your child's restrictions can actually do more harm than good.

Avoiding new foods, or anything that makes you anxious, tells your brain that the new thing is scary and worth avoiding. And the anxiety gets worse, filling the space you give it. If we avoid an unknown food and keep it as an off-limits topic or experience, our brain will build up the anxiety and magnify it over time, making it even scarier.

Anxiety is often described as a monster. Our monster grows as we feed it, and what does the anxiety monster feed on? Avoidance. The more we avoid what makes us anxious, the more that anxiety builds and the bigger the monster grows. The more we integrate scary or challenging stuff into our routine, the more familiar and comfortable it will feel. People describe routine exposure to things that cause anxiety as "forming a callus" on that anxiety. If we avoid those experiences, we prevent the "blister"—or initial, painful anxiety—from turning into a "callus."

There are several strategies you can try to stop spiraling food anxiety, but the key is to form good memories around food. We can set up their first tries of new foods for success. We can set an expectation that we have to put a little bit of each type of food on our plate. That doesn't mean we necessarily have to try it, but that everyone in our family (parents included) will have a small serving of each food on their plate. Having a very small serving of non-preferred foods can be less daunting. It makes experimentation feel safer, allowing your child to feel less anxious and more courageous.

You can also create positive food experiences outside of the dinner table. Involve your child in the entire process from start to finish. You can take them to the grocery store or to the farmer's market, or even have a garden in your backyard where they can grow fruits and vegetables. All of these places create a stress-free place for your child to learn about and explore new foods. Plus, it's fun to go shopping with your favorite adult. You can turn the trip into an adventure or a scavenger hunt—maybe, "Find foods every color of the rainbow," or, "Find two hard foods and two soft ones." Making food fun and playful is so important, and your child will feel excited to go on a quest to find new foods.

You can also involve your child in the kitchen. Have them help you mix, pour, and sort. They can watch the food cook through the oven door or help wash produce in the sink. Giving your child experiences in the kitchen will take away some of the mystery and anxiety about the food preparation process and will help them form lasting, positive memories around food.

The important factors in reducing food-related anxiety are repetition and consistency. We don't learn how to walk—or to become an adventurous eater—in one day. With lots of practice (and a bit of hard work), your child will be feeling calm, confident, and ready to explore the world of food.

30 Encouraging Positive Body Image

Almost from birth, children are exposed to all sorts of messaging about what an "ideal" body looks like and how their body shape affects their worth as a human being. No matter how hard we try to protect them from negative influences, children are constantly bombarded with information from television, magazines, billboards, the internet, and even their peers or family.

Negative body image is linked to low self-esteem, disordered eating, and depression, and these issues start way younger than we previously thought. Research suggests that children as young as three worry about being "fat" (PACEY 2016). It has been found that over 50 percent of both boys and girls between the ages of nine and fourteen are unhappy with their body shapes (PACEY 2016). Negative body image issues aren't unique to any gender, sexuality, or age, and unfortunately, everyone can fall prey to the horrible messaging from media.

There are all sorts of harmful ideals that children (and adults too) absorb, like the idea that their bodies need to be "perfect," or that there's even such thing as a "perfect" body. Negative body messaging tells them that a perfect body would give them happiness, acceptance, fulfillment, and love, so when they feel like their body doesn't match the ideal, they feel like they aren't worthy of love or acceptance. While we might not be able to prevent their exposure to damaging messages, we can give them plenty of skills to fight them.

The biggest and best way that children learn about how to feel about their bodies is through watching their parents and imitating their body image. Children are constantly watching and learning, which means that, as parents, we need to check on and monitor our own body image. There are lots of ways that we can model healthy body image.

Avoid discussing body shape and weight. This includes yourself, your children, your friends, your family, and people you see in media. That means not talking about if people (yourself included) have gained or lost weight, or if they're looking thin or fat. Instead, if you want to comment on their appearance, I suggest commenting on non-weight-related characteristics, like how happy or strong they look. This practice keeps the focus on what's most important, anyway! Like the saying goes, at the end of your life, no one will remember how much you weighed, but they'll remember what type of person you were. Reinforcing strength of character for your child can help them find meaning and value in their inner selves rather than in their physical appearance.

Model healthy eating versus dieting. Ideally, it's best for your child if you avoid strict or fad diets altogether. At the very least, you'll want to avoid discussing these in front of your children. Instead, focus on integrating healthy foods, like fruits and vegetables, into your diet in a less regimented way. It's also important not to skip meals. Instead, lead by demonstration and show your child that bodies need to eat when they're hungry. Likewise, show them that it's perfectly acceptable not to clear your plate when you're full. Teach your child to listen to their internal body cues by listening to your own body cues as well. Children learn to diet through watching their parents, and this can lead to restrictive eating, meal skipping, and all sorts of negative thoughts about their bodies and foods.

Find joy in movement. You can teach your child to love and value exercise for the way it makes their body feel rather than to burn calories or lose weight. You can teach them about how yoga lowers their stress and makes them feel strong or about how running is a great way to explore nature. Help them find a form of exercise that they enjoy. There's no wrong way to exercise, but teaching them to find the fun in strengthening themselves will help them to develop their confidence in themselves and their body. Never talk about exercise as having to "earn" that dessert or to "work off" your Thanksgiving dinner. Exercise shouldn't be a punishment but rather an expression of joy and celebration of all the wonderful things that our bodies can do. Showing your child how to value your body for what it can do, rather than what size it is, will reinforce a positive body image.

On the subject of weight, one more thing to note is that the Body Mass Index (or BMI), is a highly fallible measurement. Many people use BMI to measure if someone is over- or underweight, as it's a convenient and easy tool. That being said, the tool was invented in the 1800s, and science has come a long way since then! The BMI measurement takes into account only someone's height and weight. It doesn't account for any other factors, like how much of their weight is muscle versus fat, where they are in a growth spurt, or their bone density. Muscle weighs significantly more than fat, so a body builder may register as "obese" according to BMI scales. If you have concerns about your child's weight, discuss these with a medical professional before making judgments using their BMI. Children's bodies can take all shapes and sizes, and will likely change frequently and rapidly as they grow. Teaching your child to love the body that they're in, regardless of its size and shape, is a lesson that will last them a lifetime.

Love your own body. We've all looked in a mirror and not liked what we saw, but make sure that you aren't narrating that experience for your child. Children can read body language too, so keeping self-criticism internal includes things like not frowning at your body in the mirror. Instead, talk about what you like that your body can do. Tell them about the time that your body carried you up to the top of the mountain and you got the most beautiful view, or when your body gave you the strength to tag someone in a water balloon fight you had last year. And as the saying goes, if you can't think of anything nice to say, then don't say anything at all.

You can do everything completely right, and your child may still make a negative comment about their body. If you hear that happen, resist the instinct to dismiss it completely, like, "That's so silly—of course you're not fat." Instead, this moment can be a great learning opportunity. Take the time to discuss it with your child. Ask them where these thoughts are coming from. This conversation can give you a chance to disprove any myths they may believe about the ideal body and what their body is supposed to look like. You can emphasize that sometimes healthy bodies look different than the media would lead us to believe.

Some children may be teased for their appearance. Kids can be brutal! If you find out that this is happening, you should first take steps to stop it and validate your child and their feelings. It may help to get your child a therapist or other support to process their hurt. Even when their body image has been injured like this, with help it can bounce back and be stronger than ever.

Children are growing rapidly, and each age comes with its own body image struggles and difficulties. There are many ways that you can bolster a healthy self-image at every stage.

For babies and toddlers, it's most helpful to support their independence when possible. Toddlers are all about "doing it myself!" so setting up instances where they can be successful with new movements helps them feel strong and positive about their bodies.

Once children hit school age, they can understand a lot more about their bodies. This is a time to empower your child by teaching them about their body and how to take care of it. At this age, children like to show you what they can do! Let them! School-aged children are so proud of the new skills that they're acquiring, and they want to hear you say that you're proud of them too. This is a great time to get them involved in sports or some other form of daily active play.

As children reach puberty, they're hit with all sorts of bodily changes that can feel abrupt and surprising. Their body shapes are likely changing rapidly, they may have hair in new places, their voice may change, and more. It can feel like they don't even know their own body anymore, and these changes can take time to adjust to. There's also a lot of pressure at this age to fit in and look like their peers. During this time, you can support your child by letting them try out different looks or styles if they want to. They're trying to feel comfortable in their new body! With all their hormonal changes, their sleep patterns and weight may change quickly too. You can help them maintain a regular sleep and exercise schedule as much as possible. It can be beneficial to engage them in other activities, like volunteer work, that give them meaning and a sense of self-worth. Giving back to your family or community can help teens feel connected and valued.

Social media can have a large influence in the teenage years. Teach your child to be a discerning consumer of all media, social and otherwise. Especially in our Instagram era, show them how influencers use picture editing, angles, and lighting to change the way their body appears. Remind them that everyone's stomach has rolls when they lean forward, no matter how perfect their six-pack appears in that picture. Your teen will probably face a lot of pressure to look a certain way from social media, but you can arm them with the knowledge that real healthy bodies come in all shapes and sizes.

Having positive body image can be hard, and many adults are still unlearning a lifetime of negative body messaging. That takes a lot of patience, work, and more work. Give yourself some grace during this process too. You won't be perfect, and that's totally okay. Showing your child that it's fine to make mistakes, and that you can grow from them, will help them develop into strong, independent, and confident young adults.

31 Helping Your Child Gain Weight

While all bodies, no matter their shape or size, are worthy of value and love, sometimes children's medical teams decide that they need to gain more weight to support their growth. When this happens, it can feel tricky to tread the line between being body positive and trying to change their body. Children's heights and weights change rapidly and frequently throughout childhood, so try not to worry if you notice a brief shift in their weight. Children's bodies are often great at taking in the calories they need on their own and in their own time. If your child's medical team has decided that they could use a little extra support though, of course, follow all of their guidelines on necessary calorie intake and nutritional needs. Here are a few tips and tricks to keep in mind to make sure you're helping them continue their positive body image as you work toward their weight goals.

The first thing to do will be to work with your medical team to rule out any potential cause for your child to be underweight. Children can lose weight or have difficulty gaining weight because of a whole host of issues, including picky eating, difficulty with feeding coordination, increased energy requirements, eating disorders, or just about any other underlying disease or condition. Weight loss can be the first red flag for other conditions, so it's important to make sure that you're treating the underlying cause, if there is one. If your child's medical team has ruled out any other concerns, then it's time to start working on gaining weight at home.

When your child is underweight, it can be nerve racking and your first instinct can be to talk to everyone, including your child, about this. After all, they're the ones that need to be eating more, so why *not* tell them that they need to eat more? Pressuring your child to eat more can make them anxious, and who's hungry when they're anxious? Stress lowers our body's natural appetite, so having anxiety-inducing mealtimes can result in their eating less rather than more.

Also, talking to your child about how they're underweight can lead to negative thoughts about their body. We never want to shame our children for their bodies or draw attention to them, no matter the shape or size that they take. This includes talking to them in a seemingly positive way, like, "You look so much better now that you've put on a few more pounds." While this can sound positive, what it says to your child is, "There's a better and worse body shape to have," and, "I like you more now that your body has changed shapes," and we want our children to feel confident in any body that they have. As children get older, you can start to talk to them about ways to be healthy, including teaching them about nutrition, but try to avoid talking about their body in these conversations.

When trying to help your child gain weight, it can be easiest, healthiest, most efficient, and most cost-effective to add nutrient-rich and calorie-dense foods to their diet rather than add supplements. Some ideas for natural foods that you can add into their diets are calorie-rich items like avocado, smoothies with whole-fat yogurt, granola mix, nut butters, or hummus. You can switch their dairy products, like milk, to whole-fat if they aren't already using those.

Sometimes, while your child needs higher calorie alternatives, the rest of the family does not. In these tricky instances, I recommend finding ways to add to or modify the family meal for your child to increase their calories. For example, you could add butter to their pasta or heavy cream to their soup. You could use whole milk or yogurt in place of fat-free for their serving only. Having your child eat what the rest of the family is eating will help them to feel connected rather than singled out.

Children tend to have small stomachs, which means less food can fit in them at a time. Increasing their weight may mean more frequent meals, especially for young children. Try offering your child meals somewhere between about four to six times a day instead of the usual three to five. You can also try to keep healthy, calorie-rich snacks on hand. When we're in a rush, it's easy to default to empty-calorie snacks, like chips; that's okay some of the time. With a little bit of preparation, you can provide them with a snack that will give them a little bit more bang for their buck.

If your child goes to school, consider asking the school to track what they're eating at school. Children aren't always the best reporters on what they're eating, so sometimes it's not clear what's happening at school unless they're bringing food home. Children spend a lot of time at school though, and depending on your child's routine, they could be eating several meals there. If they're not eating well at school, that can result in a lot of missed calories. Encourage your child's teacher to check on their food intake slyly and not to draw too much attention to it or put pressure on them to eat. It can feel daunting to eat at school with all the distractions and watching peers, so we want to avoid adding any additional stressors to their schooltime routine.

Though it can feel scary to have a child who is underweight, with some consistent modifications to their mealtime routine, your child will likely gain weight in no time. As always, don't hesitate to consult with your child's medical team if you feel like you need additional support.

32 Helping Your Child Lose Weight

As noted in the previous chapter, children's weight often fluctuates during childhood, and they may regulate this on their own through their growth process. As with all medical advice, if your child's medical team has recommended that they lose weight, follow their advice on their daily calorie needs.

Regardless of your child's weight, they have a body that's worthy of love, acceptance, and celebration. According to the Centers for Disease Control, almost 20 percent of America's youth are currently classified as obese, so if your child falls into this category, they're certainly not alone (2021). The pressure to lose weight can be immense, and can quickly lead to negative body image and disordered eating if it's not carefully managed. In fact, half of all children have tried to lose weight in the past (Brown et al. 2016). A shocking 35 percent of kids have tried to do so by skipping meals, which is linked with fatigue and decreased cognitive skills. And, counterintuitively, skipping meals is correlated with a slower metabolism, which can actually make it harder to lose weight (Brown et al. 2016). Because most children don't have the tools to do it in a healthy way, trying to lose weight alone can quickly lead to unhealthy habits and disordered eating. Given the deleterious effects of disordered eating, it becomes ever more vital to help set your child up with a healthy lifestyle from the beginning.

With all routine changes for your family, it's important to start small. Making changes that are too big can cause burnout and make everyone want to give up. Developing healthy habits shouldn't be frustrating for you or for your child. Instead, we want these strategies to feel fun and manageable in the long term.

One of the best things that you can do for your child is incorporate daily active or outdoor time. The whole family can benefit from at least an hour of outdoor physical activity every day. On the weekends, start a family tradition of spending time in nature. Go enjoy a hike, or start a family soccer team. Figure out what sorts of physical activities your children like to be a part of, and participate in those with them. Being more active can be one of the best ways to strengthen their body, lose weight, and become more confident in the process.

To this end, you should limit screen and television time to one to two hours maximum for your child, if possible. Many children spend hours sitting in school each day, only to come home and sit in front of the television, computer, or another device. While we can't always control what happens at school, we can certainly limit that screen time at home. With less screen time, they'll be more likely to engage in active play at home, which can help their weight loss goals.

Another routine change that you can add is to support your child in getting an adequate amount of sleep. Children (and adults) that get less sleep are more likely to be overweight. Not getting enough sleep makes you tired, which makes it harder to be active during the day. It also increases our body's stress hormones, which signals our body to hold onto weight rather than lose it. In general, toddlers need around twelve hours of sleep, three- to six-year-olds need eleven hours, seven- to twelve-year-olds need ten hours, and teenagers need around nine hours. Helping your child maintain a good sleep routine can help them maintain a healthy weight as well.

Another idea is to have healthy snacks available for your child. When they get home from school, they're likely hungry and often head straight for the snack cabinet. It can be easy to fill up on empty calories that won't give them nutrients and will cause a sugar crash later. Instead, make sure that there's a plate of fruits or veggies out on the table when they get home. They can go straight to this for a healthy and filling snack and avoid the chips and crackers.

You can try to limit fast food by involving your children in cooking at home. Cooking can be a lot of work, and it's not always feasible between pickups and drop-offs from school, sports, and after-school activities.

When you can, though, bringing your child into the kitchen with you can teach them invaluable skills that they'll use for a lifetime. Cooking at home isn't only healthier, but it gives you more control over the portion size as well. If it feels daunting to cook every day, maybe just pick a few days a week to start out, or prepare some meals on the weekends that you can stick in the freezer for later in the week. You can have older children take some responsibility for a meal per week. Help them gather the ingredients and supervise while they get to play chef in the kitchen. They'll appreciate the chance to feel independent and develop new skills, and you'll be building healthy habits as well.

When serving your family, there are strategies that you can try to set healthy habits in place. Start by offering everyone small portions and then allow them to get additional servings if they ask for them. People of all ages are more likely to eat more food if they're presented with a larger portion size. Our brains have a harder time pausing part-way through a plate of food than they do after clearing a plate. Starting with smaller serving sizes can allow for mindfulness in choices about how much you're going to eat.

It can be hard to know what an appropriate serving size is for children. We know that it's smaller than an adult's serving size, but how small is it really? Ask your pediatrician about foods that you serve for your family frequently to get a gauge on how much you should be serving your child. This will vary with your child's age, size, and activity level. You can also serve your child on a child-sized plate as a visual reminder to use a smaller serving size. Especially when making the transition to smaller servings, children's servings can look so tiny on an adult plate. Placing the food on a smaller plate will allow it to fill up more of the plate, hopefully making the switch to smaller serving sizes a bit less frustrating. You can remind your child that they can always get additional servings if they would like.

Never make your child clear their plate if they say they're full though! Some parents want to enforce a clear plate rule to prevent food waste, but forcing your child to eat past when they're full can teach them to disregard their body cues on hunger and fullness. This can lead to overeating and is linked with obesity in adulthood. If your child doesn't want to finish their plate, that's totally okay, and you can always save the leftovers for another day.

Eating quickly is another risk factor for obesity because you eat too quickly for your body to register the cues that it's full. When you eat slowly, you give the food time to reach your stomach, and you give time for the fullness cues to transmit from your stomach to your brain. Encourage your child to eat more slowly by talking during dinner. Make dinner a time for the family to catch up and bond. Take turns telling stories, or ask your child questions about their day. Doing so will add little pauses into their meal, and will help them to more accurately tell when their stomach is full.

When talking about weight loss, people often say that you shouldn't drink your calories. This means avoiding high-calorie drinks that have less nutrition, like sugary sodas and juices. To make the transition to water easier, you can start by diluting their preferred high-calorie beverage with water. After a few weeks of diluting their juice, it will be easier to switch to plain water. If your child isn't motivated by plain water, you can make a family activity out of finding fun ways to infuse water with fruits or vegetables to make it taste good. You can add fresh fruit, lemon juice, or cucumber to your water to give it a stronger flavor. Hold a family-wide water tasting, where you take turns sipping flavored water and guessing what's in there. Rank your favorites and pack them in your family bag when you go on errands to prevent the need to stop to grab something else to drink.

As with all strategies to support your child, they'll do best if they can follow your example. You are your child's best role model. Show them the behaviors and habits that you want them to develop, and they'll pick them up. If you find that you need additional support for your child's weight loss journey, contact your physician or dietician.

Part Ten

MAINTAINING SENSORY REGULATION

Children's sensory processing is affected by many things. Some of the largest are how they eat, how they sleep, how their internal processes are functioning, and whether or not they're in any pain or discomfort.

We see this in our own bodies as adults. I always think about all the variations in my own auditory processing. On days when I haven't slept well, I want the music to be quiet on my commute to work. Loud music can feel grating and irritating. On the contrary though, when I'm well rested, I like to have the music on top volume so I can sing along. In these moments, the quiet music from my morning commute feels too quiet. Our sensory preferences and our ability to regulate our bodies change depending on where we are in our daily routine, how our nutritional needs are being met, how well-rested we are, and our internal health.

You can help your child's regulation by putting in place a consistent routine for them. When they know what to expect, their body can fall into patterns and use that consistency to assist with regulation. Consistent routines support good sleep, healthy eating habits, and regular bowel routines, all of which reinforce improved regulation (and adventurous eating!). The coming sections will provide you with problem-solving ideas on how to support your child's regulation.

33 Family Routines

A good family routine is key to success at mealtimes. With the right routine, your child will be ready to eat by the time meal and snack times roll around. There are several factors to consider when developing your family's routine.

One of the best things that you can do when structuring your daily routine is schedule your child's meals and snacks at a time when they're ready to eat and their stomachs are getting close to empty. We don't want them to be starving, though, or they'll just be cranky. Typically, when babies are born, their milk/formula schedule is determined by their hunger and by your doctor. As babies turn to toddlers and young children, scheduling their meals can get harder.

Once children fully transition onto solid foods, they typically do best with three meals and two to three snacks a day. This structure gives them enough time for their stomachs to clear and make way for new food but doesn't give them enough time to get too hungry.

You usually want to limit solid foods around two or three hours before meals, and liquids other than water, one hour before meals. This timing is about how long it takes these foods to move through their stomach. For example, it typically works well to do breakfast between seven and eight o'clock in the morning, snack between nine and ten o'clock, lunch between eleven and noon, snack between two and three in the afternoon, and then dinner between five and six o'clock. Of course, find times that work best for your family—ones that you can stay consistent with.

Be mindful about what drinks you're offering your child. Though we've touched on this before, it's important to remember that milk can be very filling and can limit children's desire to eat solid food. Try to limit milk for one to two hours before mealtimes so they're ready to eat and explore new foods when mealtime comes.

You'll also want to try to limit your child's juice intake. Juice tastes good, but it has a lot of sugar in it. This sugar can make your child feel full but doesn't provide the nutrients that they actually need. Once your child weans entirely onto solid foods, water is actually one of the best drinks that they can have. Water will keep them hydrated without giving them false feelings of fullness that limit their appetite.

Consistency is important when choosing a routine. We all have those days that get crazy, and it's impossible to stay on schedule, but overall, it's essential to have a set schedule for your child's meals. Try to pick times of day that are feasible for you to maintain on weekdays and weekends, regardless of what your schedule is. Consistency will allow them to predict when mealtime is coming and get in a mindset to eat. If a mealtime is going to change, try to talk to your children about this ahead of time. Preparing them can help prevent disruption and behavior issues.

Clear communication on transitions from activities to mealtimes can strengthen your daily routine. Give your child a five-minute warning before mealtimes. This allows them to start to wrap up whatever they're playing with and get ready for the transition to the dining table. Sometimes younger children don't have a clear understanding of what "Five more minutes!" means. If you feel like your child is having trouble with this transition, you can use a visual clock or a short hourglass so they can begin to conceptualize that length of time. A smooth mealtime transition will help them come to the table ready to eat and adventure with new foods.

You can also get your child involved prior to mealtime by having them help with shopping and food prep. There are tasks that your child can do at any age, from banging on pots and pans to mixing and pouring. Having your child be part of the food preparation process will help them be more invested in the meal. Your child can help with getting the table ready. They can set out napkins or utensils or tell other family members that the meal is ready.

During mealtime, you can support your child by being a good role model and making the dining table an enjoyable place to be. Start by thinking about what your own childhood interactions with food were like.

Consider writing down your answers to the following questions, and having any other caregivers for your child do the same. You can do this on a spare piece of paper or on the worksheet provided on New Harbinger's website for this book at http://www.newharbinger.com/49524. As you answer these questions, think about whether or not you want the answer to be the same for your children, and if not, what you need to change.

- Was mealtime fun or stressful?

- What do you like about your relationship with food, and what do you want to change?

- What are you glad you learned from your parents about food and what do you not want to pass down to your children?

- Did you eat meals together as a family or did everyone eat separately?

- Did your parents expect you to finish what was on your plate or could you leave some food?

- Did your parents offer you rewards for finishing non-preferred foods?

There are lots of factors to consider when you're thinking about what you want your children's meal experiences to be like. Again, consistency is so important. If you have a partner, discuss with them what you want your child's relationship with food to be like, and find a plan that you can both agree upon and stay consistent with.

You can be a good role model for your child by limiting distractions at mealtimes. Turn off the TV and use this as an opportunity to have good conversation with your child. Depending on how old your child is, there are lots of things you can talk about. You can talk about the colors of your food or what they taste like. You can talk about their day and what they learned at school. You can talk about what your schedule is going to be for the day. Use this as an opportunity to connect with your child and teach them about how fun the social aspect of mealtime can be.

During mealtime, try serving meals family style. Family-style meals develop children's social skills as well as their willingness to try new foods. They also help your child learn about positive mealtime behaviors.

When you're preparing your child's meal, think about choosing foods that set them up for success. Your child will be most successful with a maximum of one new or non-preferred food per meal served alongside other foods that they know and like. You can build excitement about new foods by planning some fun activities surrounding them. You could read books about new foods or, with older children, set up mealtime like a cooking or tasting competition. Hold tastings and have fun being food critics. In no time, they'll be finding fun and excitement in the process of trying a new food.

That being said, make sure your child doesn't turn you into a short-order cook. You'll save a lot of stress, money, and time by offering only one meal for the whole family. It's important that children learn that refusing food won't result in being offered whatever they want. Your child will benefit from being served what everyone else is eating.

Another way to support your child's mealtime routine is to set clear and consistent limits for them during mealtime. One of those rules should be that there's no negotiating about eating. When you plead with your child to try new foods or celebrate them when they do, they learn that they can control your attention through eating. Instead, keep the focus on having fun, being social, and taking the stress out of mealtimes. Without trying to manipulate or trick your child into eating, both you and your child will feel less stressed.

When you've decided on what you want your mealtime routine to look like, the only step left is to actually establish it! With everyone on the same page, consistency will be much easier. Some families find it helpful to write down their routine goals and to talk about this routine change with the entire family before starting. Getting your child involved in the routine-setting process will increase their willingness to go along with it.

Setting a routine and staying consistent can be *hard*. That's totally okay, and you're not alone in feeling like that. Nobody's perfect, and some days the mealtime routine will feel impossible to maintain. Give yourself some slack and know that if you ever fall off the bandwagon, you can always get back on the next day. Missing a few days here and there won't negatively affect your child as long as you return to consistency. Whenever you're maintaining your consistent routine, you're teaching your child healthy habits. Putting effort toward a good routine will help your child develop a positive relationship with food that lasts a lifetime.

34 Expanding Family Foods

It's so easy to fall into the habit of cooking the same foods day after day, especially with a picky eater. After a long day, there's not a person in the world that wouldn't feel tempted to give their child an easy food, one that they know they'll eat without a fuss. And while there's a time and a place for choosing your battles, it's important not to fall into a rut.

One easy way to insert some variety into your meals is to make sure never to feed the same food two (or ideally three) days in a row. That means, if you have chicken nuggets on Monday, you can't have them again until Wednesday. Some children can get stuck on wanting their same comfort foods over and over again. Having a rule set in place about how often you can have the same food can eliminate the fight over what to eat. You can simply tell your child, "We had that food yesterday, so we're not going to have it today." Making menu rotation a family expectation can limit the pushback your child gives you over new foods.

Another variation of this rule looks at your week as a whole. Choose one meal a day that you want to focus on increasing variety in. For many families, this is dinner, as evening is when they have the most time to cook or sit together as a family. Challenge each other to try to find one new recipe per week or month. There are lots of free, easy recipes online, and you can often limit your search based on what ingredients you're trying to include or any food limitations your family might have. It can help to schedule recipe-searching time into your week as a family routine. For example, "After Friday night dinner, we're going to spend ten minutes picking out a new recipe for next week." Meal planning can look very different from family to family, but the important thing is to be intentional and prioritize switching out your meals.

Building a family cookbook can be a great source of inspiration. When your menu planning starts to feel dry or repetitive, you'll have a collection of recipes to browse through. Your recipe collection can start small and doesn't have to be fancy. Maybe it starts as one to two recipes that your child enjoys, and you build from there. Your child can participate by writing down the name of the recipe, picking up the recipe off the printer, or cutting and gluing pictures of the meal, depending on how creative you want to be.

Other fun ways to try new recipes can start at the grocery store or farmer's market. Bring your child and pick out one new fruit, vegetable, or protein to try, and build a recipe around that. You can pick an unfamiliar food that looks interesting, or treat your shopping trip like a scavenger hunt. For example, you could say, "We need to find a vegetable that's red," and let your child help you search.

As your children get older, you can involve them in the challenge to find and try new recipes. Give your school-age children a night where they're responsible for the family meal. Maybe they can pick out or plan a meal from some choices, or you can help them search cookbooks or the internet for a new recipe. Of course, they'll need assistance with menu planning and meal preparation, but you can encourage them to take the lead on parts that they're ready to handle.

As parents, it can be easy to get stuck in our own preferences as well, and to refuse foods that we *know* we don't like. Remember though, if you want a child that's willing to be adventurous and taste new foods, you're going to need to model that behavior. You don't have to pretend that you like foods when you don't, but show them some positive ways to taste, try, and adventure through new foods. Who knows, you may end up finding a new food that you like as well!

35 Getting Everyone on the Same Page

As with most things when raising children, consistency is absolutely essential to raising an adventurous eater. That can be easier said than done, though, in circumstances where parents, guardians, and other family members disagree. Because feeding issues are so common, everyone tends to have an opinion on what's best to do for your child. Conversations about family norms and practices can end with a lot of cooks in the kitchen, so to speak.

The wonderful side of different opinions is that having multiple perspectives weighing in means that there are lots of people that care about your child. The not-so-wonderful side, of course, is that it can be difficult and frustrating to consistently follow through on the strategies that you feel are right.

This happens with divorced parents, when partners or spouses disagree, when family members help with child care, in multigenerational homes, or just when friends and family feel like they need to share their (possibly unsolicited) opinions. Who hasn't had someone offer unwanted advice about their child? With 50 percent of households containing divorced parents, and almost 20 percent of all households being multigenerational, these issues are certainly common, and there are many things that you can do to make the family dynamic flow more smoothly (Cohn and Passel 2018). Here are some strategies for those not-so-easy moments between caregivers, no matter your situation.

When parents disagree. There are so many different factors to how you feed your children that it can feel nearly impossible to agree with your partner on everything. The first step to building strategies together is to have the same information.

If your child has any medical appointments related to their feeding, it's wonderful to have both parents present. Having both parents hear any medical information firsthand can really increase investment in the process. If this doesn't apply to your child, you can still have both parents stay informed by sharing all resources, like websites or this book.

If your partner isn't willing or able to pursue outside resources, it can help to keep a list of considerations that you feel are most important. You could even put sticky notes on the book pages that you find most helpful, to try to condense the information for them. If your partner is unable to come to medical appointments, you could work together prior to the appointment to write up a list of questions that you both have. Then the partner that's able to attend the meeting can take notes on the answers to those questions, and the two of you can discuss it afterward.

Once you both have enough information to support your child, it's time for the fun part: making a plan. Start by finding common ground. What do you both feel like is going well? What can you agree needs to change? What do you like that your partner is doing, and what do they appreciate about your approach? It may even help to talk about the ways that you both were raised around food. How did your parents approach your eating as a child, and how did that make you feel? How do you feel like that has influenced you to this day?

Be careful if you find yourself falling into the trap of "this happened to me as a child and I turned out okay," when discussing your plans for your child. This argument tends to be tricky, because it's applying the outcome of your personal experience to everyone that received the same treatment that you did. Realistically, there are lots of factors into how children "turn out," and we want to do what's best for each individual child. Plus, don't we want our children to turn out better than just okay? We have a lot more research on best parenting methods available now, and it's important to consider updated information when making your parenting decisions. That's not to say that all of your parents' strategies were negative, just to make sure that you dig a little deeper if your main justification is "this is how I was raised as a child."

The two of you should work together to develop a plan that feels feasible and sustainable for you both. This will look different for every family. Some families like tackling every meal together, while some like to divvy it up so it doesn't feel overwhelming. The most important part is that you are able to consistently follow through on whatever plan the two of you develop. If you develop the plan together and both of you understand the strategies, you'll be better able to support each other and hold each other accountable.

If you find that these discussions are difficult, it can help to write down your priorities and how important they are to you prior to discussing them. The last thing that you want to do is argue in front of your child, especially during dinnertime. There are two approaches to resolving a disagreement. The first is for both parents to write down how important this issue is to them on a scale of one to ten. If this issue is a two out of ten in terms of importance for one parent and an eight out of ten for another, that's worth factoring into the discussion. The other idea is to compromise. For example, if you don't agree on having family dinner versus feeding the kids first, you might alternate nights with family dinner and couple time. Or you might agree to have a few bites of dinner all together but save the rest of your meal for after the kids are settled.

Last, you may want to plan a time to check in about a week after you institute some changes—perhaps an hour or so for the two of you to connect. How do you feel like things have been going? What's been working and what hasn't? This conversation will give you a chance to address any concerns that either of you may have before they snowball into larger issues. As you check in, remember that many strategies take at least a week or two to see a large effect.

Strategies for divorced parents (or those living apart). Extra challenges can come with your child living in multiple homes. Luckily, there are many ways that you can support your child's mealtime routine across households to ensure their success when it comes to eating!

If you and your ex-partner disagree on how best to approach your child's needs, all the strategies in the above section will still be helpful, but beyond that, there are strategies that you can implement to make the distance easier.

Parents should work together to make a plan that will function well in both households. Different homes have different needs, and both families may need to compromise to find something that will work well for everyone involved.

Keeping a food journal that goes between homes can ensure communication between each party. I normally recommend tracking what your child ate and when, as well as if there were any extra factors, like if your child had a tantrum or difficulty coming to the table at mealtime. Drop-offs and pickups can be chaotic, and it can be hard to remember everything you need to talk about. The journal helps both parents know what they missed and allows them to follow up on previous incidents that may have happened, maintaining consistency. It also makes sure that you never use your child as a messenger between you, which can foster resentment.

It can help to schedule a time into your week where the two of you can talk about everything going on with your child, feeding included. This can be a time to get on the same page, to collaborate, to solve problems, and to make a plan for the coming week. During these conversations, keep focused on your child and to maintain your child as a priority. Remember to ask your ex-partner about how they're feeling about the strategies that you've both been trying, to try to head off any potential conflicts before they escalate. It's important to keep in mind that you and your ex-partner are still a team, and you both want the best for your child, no matter what.

Depending on your custody agreement, it's possible that one parent may have significantly less time with the child and may not want to actively participate in the rule making and strategy building surrounding feeding. In these cases, it can help to make a really clear list of do's and don'ts for visitations. This keeps everyone on the same page for those shorter visits.

If you have tried absolutely everything and you can't get your ex-partner to invest in the feeding process, then you can still maintain that consistency at your home. Knowing what to expect at each home (even if the guidelines are different between homes) will still help your child feel secure in understanding the rules.

Multigenerational households. Living in a multigenerational house can be so wonderful, as it means there's no shortage of people in the house that love and care about your children. A trade-off is that all those loving people love to insist on their own parenting strategies for your child. If you all agree on how to parent your child, it can make things easier. But sometimes there are conflicts and power struggles.

Your parents did their best to raise you, so when you say that you want to try a different approach, they likely hear, "You didn't do a good enough job," and feel defensive. When your parent tells you what to do with your child, it can come across as, "I don't think you're as good of a parent as I was." This can lead to some hurt feelings for everyone involved. At the end of the day, you aren't your parents, and you each need to live your own lives and make your own decisions. You can remind your parents that every child needs different strategies, and, though you value their opinion greatly, you know your child and their needs best. If your parents or in-laws are scientifically minded, it can also be helpful to share your science and research with them, so they can participate in your strategies as well.

If you find that relations between you and your family members are getting tense, a large family meeting may help ease tensions. At this meeting, you can encourage everyone to share their own feelings and thoughts. As with every conflict, avoid using accusatory statements ("You undermined me!") and shift the focus to "I-statements" ("I felt hurt when you didn't support me in this instance"). Another common piece of advice is to stay focused on specific events rather than jump into generalizations ("You always do this!"). Following these guidelines can help keep the conversation productive and kind, rather than escalate into a larger fight.

Managing unwanted opinions from family and friends. Who hasn't gotten unwanted advice from a friend or family member? People give advice because they care and want to help, but it can be frustrating when you have a plan in place that they're disregarding. If you feel comfortable telling the unwanted advice-giver a direct "No, thank you," all the more power to you, but I know that sometimes that's easier said than done or is just impossible. In those cases, there are plenty of conflict-free ways of handling the situation.

One of the easiest things to do is to just disregard their advice. You can simply smile, nod, and go on your way. This idea works best if you have limited contact with the advice-giver. If you interact with them regularly, it may be wise to choose your battles. For example, there are some things that may not matter to you too much, like whether your child has apples or pears for snack. Giving in on smaller issues can lessen the tension with and pressure from the advice-giver. If you're close with the person giving you advice, you may also want to try educating them as well. You can quote your doctor or research to show them that your plan for your child is well thought out and supported. At the end of the day though, you are the parent and don't need permission from the advice-giver to parent your child the way you think is best.

If you feel comfortable with it, you can try talking to the advice-giver on how their advice makes you feel. You could start by reminding them that you appreciate that they care so much for your child and are trying to help, because they are! As with other issues, it's helpful to stick to "I-statements," like, "I feel uncomfortable when you tell me what to do for my child." Next, you should clearly communicate what you would like the boundaries in your relationship to be around this subject. For example, you could say, "Right now I'm comfortable with the way that we're handling things, but if I ever need advice on this subject, I'm so glad that I can go to you for help." This lets them know that you should be the one initiating the next conversation on this subject, but, hopefully, doesn't leave them with too many hurt feelings either.

Conflicts arise around parenting when all people involved care deeply about the child and their wellbeing, and all in all that's not a bad thing! It's all about finding ways to stay sane as you wade through all the solicited and not-so-solicited advice out there. You know what's best for your child, and deserve to have your loved ones support the plan that's best for them.

36 Tips for Dining Out

No one wants the experience of packing everybody into the car, driving out to the restaurant, and sitting down to order, only to have your child have a meltdown or get up and start running around. While dining out can be a great opportunity to try new foods or spend time together as a family, it can certainly be stressful too. Luckily, there are lots of tips you can try to set your child up for success.

The first thing to do is to choose a good day for going out to eat. Find a day when your child is well rested and healthy. A tired or sick child is already set to be cranky and irritable.

You'll also want to remember to bring whatever supplies you may need. If your child has a particular cup or utensil that they prefer, you can bring those. A bit of familiarity can go a long way at a new restaurant.

That being said, I encourage families not to bring electronics when going out to eat. While effective in distracting children, electronics also limit their engagement in the meal and the social interaction that goes along with it. They keep their attention on the device and not on the food in front of them, which prevents them from really engaging with and learning about their food.

If going out to eat is a known stressor in your family, another thing you'll want to be intentional about is which restaurant you're choosing. Pick somewhere that's a close drive. Going for a long drive in the car can be stressful and exhausting on its own, and expecting your child to be able to hold it together for a drive *and* a meal can be a bit much.

If you don't live close to a family-friendly restaurant, you may consider finding one with a park nearby instead. You can combine the trip, going first to the park to let your child run off some extra steam, and then to the restaurant. Once your child has had a chance to play and work up an appetite, they may be more willing to sit with you for a meal out in public.

I recommend finding a restaurant where you know that your picky eater can find *something* safe to order. If they feel overwhelmed by the menu, they'll likely show that in their behaviors. Knowing that they have something safe to order will give them confidence and make it more likely that they'll be willing to participate in the whole meal (and maybe even try a bite of a new food!).

Many children choose dining out as a time to display all their worst behaviors because they think that the behavior modification strategies that their parents use at home won't get used while at a restaurant. Lots of parents are good at not feeding into their children's naughty behavior at home, but it can be embarrassing out in public, and it's tempting to give in to their demands to keep them behaving. Unfortunately though, children are smart and pick up on this, and many won't hesitate to use it to their advantage, upping their demands each time. If you can show your child that you have the same behavior expectations and strategies while at a restaurant as at home, they'll be less likely to misbehave.

All guests deserve to be able to enjoy their meal in peace. For this reason, keep your child's behaviors in mind when practicing going out to eat. Maybe pick off-peak times, when you know there won't be many other guests to disrupt if your child starts to act out. It can also be beneficial to ask for a table in a back corner, away from other people, or to choose a restaurant that has an outdoor section. If your child is unable to manage their behaviors inside, think about taking a quick break outside to let them calm down before returning inside. For many children, a short recess is enough to regroup and continue to participate in mealtime.

If you've picked some good places to practice and you're still having a hard time, it can be helpful to do a bit more to prepare your child prior to going. Talk to them about restaurants and what they can expect. Depending on their age, you can look at the menu together, talk about eating at restaurants, or read stories and watch videos about what dining out can be like.

Last, but certainly not least, if you feel overwhelmed and things seem to be going downhill, don't be afraid to call it quits and try again another day. Everyone has bad days, children included, and it's okay to head home early and enjoy your meal at home instead. Give yourself permission to give it another try on another day. Just don't give up entirely. Children are always learning new skills, and with adequate preparation and practice, they'll end up surprising you. If it's not today, one day soon, you and your child will be able to enjoy a meal out together.

37 Tips for Holidays

There's a lot of pressure on everyone around the holidays or other family gatherings. From the parents' perspective, we want our child to reflect well on us in front of other family members, we want to have a peaceful celebration, and we want to focus on enjoying the holiday without worry. From our kids' perspective, they may be in a new environment, or surrounded by people they aren't as familiar with who want to cuddle with them. They might be wearing a new outfit that's itchy or uncomfortable. They might be eating at a time that's outside their routine, or changing their schedule altogether. The gathering might be noisy or distracting, and let's be honest, many gatherings involve family bickering, which can be stressful or scary. When we add all these pressures to a routine that's already stressful to begin with, it can throw our kids over the top. So how do you set your child up for success?

The key to any good plan is successful preparation. Talk to your child about the upcoming holiday *before* you're on your way there. One or two weeks in advance, start talking about the holiday and what it might entail. Talk about whose house you're going to, what people will be there, and what you might be eating. Letting your child know what to expect helps mitigate the anxiety they might feel around the day.

It can also help to set some clear expectations for the day. You can talk about rules that might be different in a new house. Maybe you're going to Grandma's house, and she has a dog that doesn't want to be petted, or maybe you're going to Uncle's house, and his indoor plants aren't allowed to be touched. New situations can bring up behavioral questions for your child, and you can help prevent outbursts by giving them some structure on what to expect and what's expected of them.

For a picky eater, the meal can be the most stressful piece, but luckily, there's lots that you can do to get them ready. One thing that you can do is to prepare a food to bring with you. That's not to say to bring a special meal just for them. Rather, bring one side dish for everyone to share. Allowing your child to be part of the meal preparation is an important step in helping them to feel comfortable, but that can be hard when you're going to someone else's house for a meal. Bringing one piece of the meal will give them one "safe" food that they can use as a jumping off point for trying other foods at the gathering.

Another tactic to keep in mind is finding ways to practice and prepare for the other foods that will be there. Lots of holidays have their own special foods that go along with them, and we don't often prepare those foods at other times of the year. We have to remember, though, that it can take twenty or forty times of trying a food before we feel comfortable with it. If they're trying it for the first time at this party, it will be difficult to have success! While it can be extra work to prepare these special foods outside of holiday time, your child will feel much more confident if they're being served foods that they've tried before rather than brand-new ones at the gathering.

Before the holiday, you can also set you and your child up for success by setting expectations with your other family members. Older family members love and care about your child a lot, and they often have their own ideas about how to parent. While they mean well, they don't know as much as you do about the things that your child has been working on, the strategies you have in place, or what's important to your family during mealtimes. Their well-meaning attempts to encourage your child to eat can actually increase stress rather than decrease it. By getting conversations about mealtime expectations out of the way before the holiday— rather than during—you can avoid exposing your child to unhelpful opinions. It helps to remind family that you have a plan and are doing research and taking active steps to meet your child's needs. Learning to be an adventurous eater is a marathon, not a sprint, and it can take time. Sometimes these extra reminders can help your loving family members remember your family's priorities around food and respect those boundaries that you set up.

Although a holiday meal is different and special, make sure to keep up a lot of the strategies that we've discussed earlier in this book to set your child up for success. Aim to put one to two new foods on their plate and fill the rest with familiar foods. Your child will be more likely to branch out and try one or two new foods than they would be if their entire plate was full of new foods.

Also, keep the meal length to around twenty minutes. Everyone loves to sit and chat during family gatherings, and mealtimes can extend for several hours in some families. While it would be great if your child could join for all of that, they're likely not ready to do so from a developmental standpoint. Keep your expectations to the normal twenty minutes. After twenty minutes, it's understandable that your child would want and need to get up from the table, and you should allow them to do so if possible.

After the meal, it can help for them to have a safe space to calm down if they need it. Family mealtimes, while fun, can be overwhelming and a bit daunting for picky eaters, and they may need to get away from it all. See if the host has a quiet room in the back where they'll let your child retreat when they need it. Having a peaceful place to go can empower them to be braver during mealtimes because they know if they overextend themselves, they'll be able to recharge.

Last, but certainly not least, remember to save some leftovers for practicing later at home! Regardless of your child's readiness for bravery at this year's holiday, getting in some extra practice with those special holiday foods will set them up for more success next year.

38 Tips for Eating at School

While your child probably loves going to school, lunchtime can be extra stressful for picky eaters. Lunchtime at school is typically pretty short, and there's a lot of pressure on your child to eat. Your child may also be overwhelmed by the number of children in their space.

While lunchtime can be fun for children that are confident eaters, the pressure can be overwhelming for those that are feeling a bit more nervous. This can lead to decreased appetite and willingness to try new foods. You may find that your child is only willing to eat their very favorite things at school, or they may not be willing to eat at all. There are several things that you can do to support your child in feeling comfortable eating in this environment.

The first thing that you're going to want to do is learn a little bit more about your child's lunchtime experience at school. Depending on your child's age, you can talk to them about this or you can ask their school directly for more information:

- How much time are they given?

- Where do they eat?

- What's the noise level like and whom do they sit with?

- Is lunch right before recess? Sometimes children like to skip lunch to be able to get to the fun part—playing on the playground!

It can also help to think a little bit about your child's food preferences:

- Does temperature play a role in their enjoyment of certain foods?

- Is your child able to confidently open their food containers independently, or do they need help?

Once you have all the answers you need, you can work with your child to develop a plan.

It can also be helpful to ask your child what they see as barriers to successful mealtimes at school. Why do they think their lunchbox is coming back home full? You may be surprised at your child's insights. Often they know exactly what's going on and just haven't shared it with you yet.

Some families like to find a weekend and practice packing a meal to eat at home or out at a picnic. If the trial meal goes smoothly at home, then you know that the problem is around the eating experience at school, and not about the food itself. If not, you may be able to tease out what it is about the food that they're not enjoying. Perhaps there's a way to modify the temperature, texture, or accessibility of the food after it has been stored in the lunchbox.

During this trial run, you can have your child help you pack what they think would be a good lunchtime meal. Try making a game out of finding fun lunchtime meals to get your child more invested in the process. You can have them aim to get as many different-colored foods in their lunch as possible or even have them come up with different presentations of familiar foods, like using cookie cutters on their sandwiches or apple slices.

When choosing foods for your child's lunch, keep in mind that the best time to introduce new foods is when the child feels rested, regulated, comfortable, and safe. Lunchtime at school is usually not that time. Typically, children are feeling very excited (or maybe overwhelmed) at lunch, and surprising them with unfamiliar food doesn't set them up for success in trying new things. Save the new foods for at home, and once they've tried them a time or two at home, they'll be ready to add them to their lunch at school. It can also help to think outside the box and choose a variety of foods for their lunches, rather than pack the same thing each day. Having variety in their lunch will significantly decrease the odds that they grow tired of those foods. Scheduling changes to their typical lunch menu ahead of time can let your child know what to expect so that they're not guessing at what's in their lunchbox.

Once they've packed up their lunch for your trial run, they can store it as they normally store it at school, whether that's in the fridge or somewhere else with an icepack. This will help simulate the school lunch experience as well as possible. When it comes time for lunch, observe your child eating. You'll be able to see how they're doing. This will also give you a chance to check out what their lunch looks like after being packed up all day. Maybe their sandwich is getting crushed, or their fruit is mushy. Little things like their foods' appearance can have a big effect on children's willingness to eat.

The next step will be to look at how the environment of the lunchroom is affecting your child. It may be helpful to talk to the teacher to educate them as to how they can best support your child during lunch. Some children prefer to be left alone while eating, and some prefer to have someone check in on them to remind them what a great job they're doing and how brave they are while they eat. Your child may be overwhelmed by the noise or number of people watching them. It's possible that there's a quieter area of the room where they can eat, or a smaller table. If those aren't options, they could position themselves facing away from the majority of the room so they feel less pressured. There are lots of ways to help make the lunchroom feel more like the comfort of home.

If purchasing school lunch is best for your family, there are still steps that you can take to set them up for success. Talk to them about the process of purchasing food. Are they feeling confident with how to do that? Do they know the cafeteria workers and do they feel comfortable with them? You'll want to ask your school for a copy of the lunch meal schedule. This way, you can talk with your child about what foods are going to be available so they can prepare themselves. You can also try to scope out which types of foods they'll feel most confident with.

If you want to transition your child from bringing to buying lunch, or vice versa, you'll want to start slowly. Start by having them try the new system out one day a week, and then increase it from there. This will allow them to get comfortable with the change in routine before the pressure is on full time.

Last, it's important to keep a routine even on days when your child isn't at school. Maintaining a set time and routine for lunch on the weekends will set your child up for success when they return to school on Monday.

Conclusion: The Start of a Lifelong Food Adventure

Congratulations! By finishing this book, you've taken a huge step toward improving your family's relationship with food, and hopefully, you're well on your way to enjoying every mealtime with your child.

You've learned how to understand and support your child's sensory systems to set your child up for success at home and in the community, how to modify your family routines, how to structure your mealtimes, and how to involve your children in the whole process. You have some ideas for problem-solving through tricky behaviors, and you're ready to face future challenges that come your way.

It's important to remember that making huge changes like these can take time. It's a marathon and not a sprint! Negative habits likely took years to develop and grow stronger, which means that they'll take some time to break down as well. With practice and intentionality, you can speed up the process of breaking picky eating habits and will see frequent and regular positive changes moving forward.

If you've tried all these strategies and are still feeling stuck or like it's too much to manage, there are plenty of feeding therapists that will help guide you through the steps. Don't hesitate to reach out to your pediatrician or other local resources for a referral to feeding therapy. Making positive changes to your family's eating routine and relationship with food can take work, but the benefits are immeasurable.

Acknowledgments

This book has been such a group effort, and there are so many people without whom this book would not exist.

I owe a huge thanks to my agent, Rita Rosenkranz, for believing in this project from the beginning, and for encouraging me through rewrites to shape it into what it is today. You saw a vision for my book even before I did, and I am grateful for your endless support to help it get there.

I am enormously grateful to the large team at New Harbinger for taking on my manuscript, and for the countless hours of work that you've poured into it. An extra-large thank you to Elizabeth Hollis Hansen for advocating for this project and what it could be.

I owe an enormous debt to my friends and colleagues for their constant support and for inspiring me to be the best clinician that I can be. I am so thankful that I get to continually learn from you all and to be inspired by the amazing work that you do.

I have endless love and gratitude for my husband, Parker, who was absolutely integral to the development of this book. Thank you for tirelessly helping me read and edit every rewrite (of which there were *many*), and for always believing in this project and cheering me on every step of the way. Your support and love mean the world to me.

Last, a huge thank you to the families and patients that I work with. You are a constant inspiration to me, and I am so grateful for the opportunity to be a small part of this season in your lives.

Glossary

adaptive anxiety: A body's leveled response to keep you safe in times of danger.

bolus: A ball of chewed food in your mouth.

disordered anxiety: Anxious feelings that disrupt your life and aren't proportionate to your level of safety.

food repertoire: List of foods that your child is willing to eat.

gross motor movements: Movements that use large muscles in our torso, arms, or legs. Examples include running, jumping, climbing, and more.

interoceptive sense: Sensory system responsible for internal cues, like hunger and thirst.

olfactory: Related to a sense of smell.

pocketing: Holding food in your mouth without swallowing.

proprioceptive sense: Sensory system responsible for body awareness and motor planning.

sensory input: The stimulation of one of our senses. Things that are more stimulating provide more input than those that are less stimulating.

sensory processing: How the body organizes sensation from one's own body and the environment, making it possible to use the body effectively within the environment.

vestibular sense: Sensory system responsible for balance.

Additional Resources

Cadwell, K. 2007. "Latching-On and Suckling of the Healthy Term Neonate: Breastfeeding Assessment. *Journal of Midwifery & Women's Health* 52(6): 638–42.

Chen, W.G., D. Schloesser, A.M. Arensdorf, J.M. Simmons, C. Cui, R. Valentino, J.W. Gnadt, L. Nielsen, C. St. Hillaire-Clarke, V. Spruance, T.S. Horowitz, et al. 2021. "The Emerging Science of Interoception: Sensing, Integrating, Interpreting, and Regulating Signals Within the Self. *Trends in Neurosciences* 44(1): 3–16.

Cojocaru, M., S. Millard, and S. Stevenson. 2018. "Serving Fruits and Vegetables in Kid-Friendly Shapes Increased Fruit and Vegetable Consumption in Preschool Children Aged 2-5 Years." *Loma Linda University Research Reports*, 18. https://scholarsrepository.llu.edu/rr/18.

Dunn, W. 1997. "The Impact of Sensory Processing Abilities on the Daily Lives of Young Children and Their Families: A Conceptual Model. *Infants and Young Children* 9: 23–35.

Engel-Yeger, B., R. Hardal-Nasser, and E. Gal. 2015. "The Relationship Between Sensory Processing Disorders and Eating Problems Among Children with Intellectual Developmental Deficits." *British Journal of Occupational Therapy* 79(1): 17–25.

Fishbein, M., S. Cox, C. Swenny, C. Mogren, L. Walbert, and C. Fraker. 2006. "Food Chaining: A Systematic Approach for the Treatment of Children with Feeding Aversion." *Nutrition in Clinical Practice* 21(2): 182–4.

Lafraire, J., C. Rioux, A. Giboreau, and D. Picard. 2016. "Food Rejections in Children: Cognitive and Social/Environmental Factors Involved in Food Neophobia and Picky/Fussy Eating Behavior. *Appetite* 96: 347–57.

Larsen, J. K., R.C.J. Hermans, E.F.C. Sleddens, R.C.M.E. Engels, J.O. Fisher, and S.P.J. Kremers. 2015. "How Parental Dietary Behavior and Food Parenting Practices Affect Children's Dietary Behavior. Interacting Sources of Influence?" *Appetite* 89: 246–257. https://doi.org/10.1016/j.appet.2015.02.012

Lindberg, L., G. Bohlin, and B. Hagekull. 1991. "Early Feeding Problems in a Normal Population." *International Journal of Eating Disorders* 10(4): 395–405.

Loth, K., S. Friend, M. Horning, D. Neumark-Sztainer, and J. Fulkerson. 2016. "Directive and Non-Directive Food-Related Parenting Practices: Associations Between an Expanded Conceptualization of Food-Related Parenting Practices and Child Dietary Intake and Weight Outcomes." *Appetite* 107: 188–95. https://doi.org/10.1016/j.appet.2016.07.036

Mason, T. B. 2015. "Parental Instrumental Feeding, Negative Affect, and Binge Eating Among Overweight Individuals." *Eating Behaviors* 17: 107–10. https://doi.org/10.1016/j.eatbeh.2015.01.013.

Michel, C., C. Velasco, E. Gatti, and C. Spence. 2014. "A Taste of Kandinsky: Assessing the Influence of the Artistic Visual Presentation of Food on the Dining Experience." *Flavour* 3: 7. https://doi.org/10.1186/2044-7248-3-7.

Moray, J., A. Fu, K. Brill, and M.S. Mayoral. 2007. "Viewing Television While Eating Impairs the Ability to Accurately Estimate Total Amount of Food Consumed." *Bariatric Nursing and Surgical Patient Care* 2(1): 71–6.

Nadon, G., D.E. Feldman, W. Dunn, and E. Gisel. 2011. "Association of Sensory Processing and Eating Problems in Children with Autism Spectrum Disorders." *Autism Research and Treatment* 541926.

Reilly S, D. Skuse, and X. Poblete. 1996. "Prevalence of Feeding Problems and Oral Motor Dysfunction in Children with Cerebral Palsy: A Community Survey." *The Journal of Pediatrics* 129(6): 877–82. DOI: 10.1016/s0022-3476(96)70032-x.

Renner, B., G. Sproesser, F.M. Stok, and H. Schupp. 2016. "Eating in the Dark: A Dissociation Between Perceived and Actual Food Consumption." *Food Quality and Preference* 50: 145-51.

Roberts, L., J.M. Marx, and D.R. Musher-Eizenman. 2018. "Using Food as a Reward: An Examination of Parental Reward Practices." *Appetite* 120: 318–26. https://doi.org/10.1016/j.appet.2017.09.024.

Robinson, E., P. Aveyard, A. Daley, K. Jolly, A. Lewis, D. Lycett, and S. Higgs. 2013. "Eating Attentively: A Systematic Review and Meta-Analysis of the Effect of Food Intake Memory and Awareness on Eating." *The American Journal of Clinical Nutrition* 97(4): 728–42.

Shaw, S. M., and R. Martino. 2013. "The Normal Swallow: Muscular and Neurophysiological Control." *Otolaryngologic Clinics of North America* 46(6): 937–56.

Spence, C., B. Piqueras-Fiszman, C. Michel, O. Deroy. 2014. "Plating manifesto (II): The Art and Science of Plating." *Flavour* 3(1): 1–12.

Sullivan, P. B., B. Lambert, M. Rose, M. Ford-Adams, A. Johnson, and P. Griffiths. 2000. "Prevalence and Severity of Feeding and Nutritional Problems in Children with Neurological Impairment: Oxford Feeding Study." *Developmental Medicine & Child Neurology* 42(10): 674–80.

Thompson, S. D., D.A. Bruns, and K.W. Rains. 2010. "Picky Eating Habits or Sensory Processing Issues? Exploring Feeding Difficulties in Infants and Toddlers." *Young Exceptional Children* 13(2): 71–85.

Tuthill, J.C., and E. Azim. 2018. "Proprioception." *Current Biology* 28(5): R194-203.

Zellner, D.A., E. Siemers, V. Teran, R. Conroy, M. Lankford, A. Agrafiotis, L. Ambrose, and P. Locher. 2011. "Neatness Counts. How Plating Affects Liking for the Taste of Food." *Appetite* 57(3): 642–8.

References

American Academy of Pediatrics. 2011. *Bright Futures: 3rd Edition Pocket Guide*, edited by Katrina Holt. https://brightfutures.aap.org/Bright %20Futures%20Documents /BFNutrition3rdEdPocketGuide.pdf.

Braden, A., K. Rhee, C.B. Peterson, S.A. Rydell, N. Zucker, and K. Boutelle. 2014. "Associations Between Child Emotional Eating and General Parenting Style, Feeding Practices, and Parent Psychopathology." *Appetite* 80: 35–40. https://doi.org/10.1016/j .appet.2014.04.017.

Brown, C.L., J.A. Skelton, E.M. Perrin, and A.C. Skinner. 2016. "Behaviors and Motivations for Weight Loss in Children and Adolescents. *Obesity* 24(2): 446–52. https://doi.org/10.1002/oby.21370.

Bryant-Waugh, R., L. Markham, R.E. Kreipe, and B.T. Walsh. 2010. "Feeding and Eating Disorders in Childhood." *International Journal of Eating Disorders* 43(2): 98–111.

Carruth, B.R., and J.D. Skinner. 2000. "Revisiting the Picky Eater Phenomenon: Neophobic Behaviors of Young Children." *Journal of the American College of Nutrition* 19(6): 771–80.

Centers for Disease Control and Prevention. "Childhood Obesity Facts." Last reviewed April 5, 2021. Accessed September 24, 2021. https:// www.cdc.gov/obesity/data/childhood.html.

Cohn, D., and J.S. Passel. 2018. "Record 64 Million Americans Live in Multigenerational Households." Pew Research Center. April 5, 2018. https://www.pewresearch.org/fact-tank/2018/04/05/a-record-64 -million-americans-live-in-multigenerational-households/.

Edwards, K.L., J.M. Thomas, S. Higgs, and J. Blissett. 2022. "Exposure to Models' Positive Facial Expressions Whilst Eating a Raw Vegetable Increases Children's Acceptance and Consumption of the Modelled Vegetable." *Appetite* 168: 105779.

Fraker, C., M. Fishbein, S. Cox, and L. Walbert. 2007. *Food Chaining: The Proven 6-step Plan to Stop Picky Eating, Solve Feeding Problems, and Expand Your Child's Diet.* Cambridge, MA: Da Capo Lifelong Books.

Harris L.A., S. Hansel, J. DiBaise J, M.D. Crowell. 2006. "Irritable Bowel Syndrome and Chronic Constipation: Emerging Drugs, Devices, and Surgical Treatments. *Curr Gastroenterol Rep.* 8 (4): 282–90.

Nehring, I., T. Kostka, R. von Kries, and E.A. Rehfuess. 2015. "Impacts of In Utero and Early Infant Taste Experiences on Later Taste Acceptance: A Systematic Review." *The Journal of Nutrition* 145(6): 1271–9.

Nekitsing, C., P. Blundell-Birtill, J.E. Cockroft, and M.M. Hetherington. 2018. "Systematic Review and Meta-Analysis of Strategies to Increase Vegetable Consumption in Preschool Children Aged 2–5 Years." *Appetite* 127: 138–54.

Pfeffer, A.J. "'Stop Eating…Clean Your Plate!': The Effects of Parental Control of Food Consumption During Childhood on College Females' Eating Behavior." PhD diss., Texas A&M University, 2009.

Professional Association for Childcare and Early Years. 2016. "Children as Young as 3 Unhappy with Their Bodies." August 31, 2016. https://www.pacey.org.uk/news-and-views/ news/views/archive/2016-news /august-2016/children-as-young-as-3-unhappy-with-their-bodies/.

Robinson, E., P. Aveyard, and S.A. Jebb. 2015. "Is Plate Clearing a Risk Factor for Obesity? A Cross-Sectional Study of Self-Reported Data in US Adults." *Obesity* 23(2): 301–4. https://doi.org/10.1002/oby.20976.

Robinson, E., and C.A. Hardman. 2016. "Empty Plates and Larger Waists: A Cross-Sectional Study of Factors Associated with Plate Clearing Habits and Body Weight." *European Journal of Clinical Nutrition* 70(6): 750–2.

Satter, E. 1990. "The Feeding Relationship: Problems and Interventions. *The Journal of Pediatrics* 117(2): S181–9.

Satter, Ellyn. 2000. *Child of Mine: Feeding with Love and Good Sense.* Boulder, CO: Bull Pub.

Zampollo, F., K.M. Kniffin, B. Wansink, and M. Shimizu. 2012. "Food Plating Preferences of Children: The Importance of Presentation on Desire for Diversity." *Acta Paediatrica* 101(1): 61–6.

Zickgraf, H.F., and A. Elkins. 2018. "Sensory Sensitivity Mediates the Relationship Between Anxiety and Picky Eating in Children/ Adolescents Ages 8–17, and in College Undergraduates: A Replication and Age-Upward Extension." *Appetite* 128: 333–9.

Lara Dato, MS, OTR/L, is a pediatric occupational therapist with a specialty certification in feeding, eating, and swallowing—one of approximately fifty professionals with these credentials in the US. In addition to years as a feeding therapist, she has taught courses on feeding therapy across the country. Her passion is helping picky eaters and their families find joy in adventurous eating!

Foreword writer **Suzanne Mouton-Odum, PhD,** is a licensed psychologist who has helped children and families manage anxiety and difficult behaviors for more than twenty years. She coauthored *Psychological Interventions for Children with Sensory Dysregulation* and *Helping Your Child with Sensory Regulation* with Ruth Goldfinger Golomb.

Foreword writer **Ruth Goldfinger Golomb, LCPC,** is senior clinician, supervisor, and codirector of the training program at the Behavior Therapy Center of Greater Washington, where she has worked for more than thirty years.

Real change *is* possible

For more than forty-five years, New Harbinger has published proven-effective self-help books and pioneering workbooks to help readers of all ages and backgrounds improve mental health and well-being, and achieve lasting personal growth. In addition, our spirituality books offer profound guidance for deepening awareness and cultivating healing, self-discovery, and fulfillment.

Founded by psychologist Matthew McKay and Patrick Fanning, New Harbinger is proud to be an independent, employee-owned company. Our books reflect our core values of integrity, innovation, commitment, sustainability, compassion, and trust. Written by leaders in the field and recommended by therapists worldwide, New Harbinger books are practical, accessible, and provide real tools for real change.

newharbingerpublications

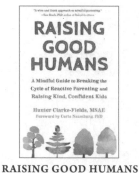
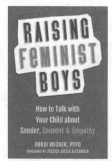
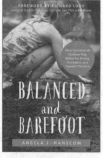
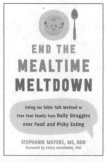
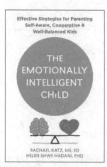
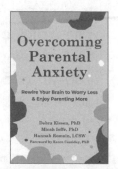

Did you know there are **free tools** you can download for this book?

Free tools are things like **worksheets, guided meditation exercises**, and **more** that will help you get the most out of your book.

You can download free tools for this book— whether you bought or borrowed it, in any format, from any source—from the New Harbinger website. All you need is a NewHarbinger.com account. Just use the URL provided in this book to view the free tools that are available for it. Then, click on the "download" button for the free tool you want, and follow the prompts that appear to log in to your NewHarbinger.com account and download the material.

You can also save the free tools for this book to your **Free Tools Library** so you can access them again anytime, just by logging in to your account! Just look for this button on the book's free tools page.

+ Save this to my free tools library

If you need help accessing or downloading free tools, visit **newharbinger.com/faq** or contact us at **customerservice@newharbinger.com**.